Colin Rose is Managing Director of Uni-Vite Ltd.
and is a graduate of the London School of
Economics. He worked in marketing for various
major companies before becoming co-founder of
an advertising company. In 1974, he formed
Topaz Publishing, based in the Buckinghamshire
village of Great Missenden. In the course of his
publishing research, he came upon the concept of
VLCDs.

Malcolm Nicholl is Marketing Director of
Uni-Vite Ltd., and is a former journalist with 14
years experience working for local and national
newspapers in both Britain and the USA. A front
page article which he wrote sparked the interest
in very low calorie diets in the States leading to
more than 5,000,000 Americans following such
slimming plans.

The Amazing Micro Diet

MALCOLM J. NICHOLL AND COLIN ROSE

SPHERE BOOKS LIMITED
London and Sydney

First published in Great Britain by
Sphere Books Ltd., 1985
Reprinted 1985
Copyright © Malcolm J. Nicholl and Colin Rose, 1985
30–32 Gray's Inn Road, London WC1X 8JL

TRADE
MARK

Set in 10/11pt Linotron Times

Printed and bound in Great Britain by
Cox & Wyman Ltd, Reading

CONTENTS

FOREWORD

By Victor Wynn, MD, FRCP, F.R.C. Path., Professor of Human Metabolism, St Mary's Hospital, London University.

This book is about Very Low Calorie Diets in general and one particular brand, The Uni-Vite Micro Diet.

This diet is effectively a diet of 330–500 calories which was formulated to include all the nutrients the slimmer needs, except the calories. The theory is that weight loss will be fast and encouraging, but the slimmer will be well because he or she is receiving all the necessary nutrition.

Research on Very Low Calorie Diets (VLCDs) dates back 30 years or more and there is no question that they are effective. I would concur with the conclusion of the largest expert survey on the subject by experienced American physicians Drs Wadden, Stunkard and Brownell that 'the most important recent development in the medical treatment of obesity is the widespread use of Very Low Calorie Diets'.

I was not always so sure. I originally felt that the best way of treating obesity was the conventional approach, by which I mean an 800–1,000-calorie diet. My own work and observation have led me to conclude that for many over-weight people the Very Low Calorie Diet is indeed an excellent answer to long-term weight loss. Of course, training in better eating habits and healthier methods of cooking are also important in the long-term management of obesity.

I am aware that the subject of VLCDs is controversial. There is a debate on the minimum level of protein that is adequate and debate on whether VLCDs should be available to the general public without close, even hospital, medical supervision. My own studies, and the fact that there have been very extensive clinical trials on VLCDs, encompassing over 10,000 people, lead me to conclude that:

1. The level of daily protein provided by the specific Very Low Calorie Diet food discussed in this book is adequate for the recommended periods of use

and

2. Given the supervision of the General Practitioner concerned, and given that the contra indications and instructions on the pack are strictly observed, well formulated Very Low Calorie Diets are safe for use in a normal work and home environment.

I have myself observed patients who, under hospital conditions, have been using a 650-calorie diet continually for several months at a time. They were fit and well and showed no sign of protein depletion which is the general concern of those who question the widespread use of VLCDs. In practice patients need the encouragement of a satisfying rapid rate of weight loss at the beginning of the diet. *Then*, when they have lost the weight, they have the motivation to change their lifestyle to healthier eating.

In short, I believe that a VLCD programme like the Micro Diet programme is a much needed and realistic answer to the problem of obesity.

Publisher's Note

Although the publishers are confident that the opinions and advice in this book are based upon well-documented clinical evidence, they would like to point out that Very Low Calorie Diets are unsuitable for certain people. Anyone planning to use The Micro Diet should consult their doctor. To encourage this the authors have provided, in Chapter 5, a questionnaire and, in Appendix B, a letter for your doctor outlining the facts.

The publishers have made every effort to ensure that none of the advice contained in this book could be damaging to health but they can accept no responsibility for effects upon anybody following The Micro Diet. Readers are reminded that the authors' recommended nutrition intake, daily fluid consumption and medical advice are important and should be followed strictly.

INTRODUCTION

'Make the flab vanish with Micro Magic'. That was how Britain's best-selling daily newspaper, the *Sun*, trumpeted the sweeping successes enjoyed by thousands of slimmers on The Micro Diet.

'The Miracle Micro Diet', proclaimed the somewhat smaller *Darlington Evening Despatch* just as exuberantly; while headlines such as 'Micro Diet aids inch war' and 'New way to beat the bulge', have been commonplace.

In just two years The Micro Diet has raced to the top of the slimming popularity stakes, with more than half a million users in Britain alone. It has overcome the initial scepticism of health professionals and 'seasoned' dieters for whom all other methods have failed. Because it works.

The concept behind the plan is blindingly simple: to provide the body with all essential nutrients without those fattening calories. The goal: fastest possible weight loss without jeopardising the health and well-being of the slimmer.

In the past dietitians have had little option but to recommend a minimum daily intake of 1,000 calories because, with ordinary solid food, they could not guarantee the full nutritional requirements in anything less. In fact, many of the 1,000-calorie a day plans, promoted so enthusiastically by the various health organisations, diet clubs and slimming magazines, do not contain all of the recommended daily amounts of vital nutrients. This is not a criticism, simply a statement of fact. The body needs something like 50 essential nutrients, amino acids, vitamins, minerals and trace elements. To devise a daily menu that incorporates every one of them, in the recom-

1

mended amounts, is difficult. To devise a menu that contains all of them in just 1,000 calories of ordinary food is *extremely* difficult.

In the last two decades, thanks to the development of the micro chip, the scientific boffins have miniaturised computers to such an extent that a computer which would have filled a room, now sits handily on a desktop. Calculators the size of credit cards and wristwatch televisions have even been developed. In exactly the same way, the food scientists have 'miniaturised' all of the nutrients you need on a weight loss plan into just 330 calories a day. To the medical profession it's known as a Very Low Calorie Diet. We call it The Micro Diet – for obvious reasons.

Every single day's meals provide all of the protein, carbohydrate and essential fatty acids as well as every single vitamin, mineral, trace element and electrolyte. (An electrolyte is an element like sodium, potassium, chloride. A daily intake of electrolytes is needed; a deficiency can cause tiredness and irregular heart beats.) All the nutrients recommended by leading health authorities in only 330 calories. And it's done, not by roaming the rows of a supermarket, painstakingly picking and choosing items from the shelves, but simply by mixing a powdered formula with water. In this ultimate weight loss plan the dieter helps herself to three servings, of just 110 calories each, and drinks plenty of water. And that's it!

Despite the very low calorie level, you are likely to feel fully satisfied. Because of the very low calorie level most people lose weight very rapidly – the average is 16–20 pounds a month. And with a weight loss plan that has undergone more clinical testing than any other slimming method available today.

We first came across the concept in an international medical journal. Frankly, we were sceptical. The scientific evidence seemed beyond reproach, but firmly entrenched in our minds was that traditional dietary myth: the body needs at least 1,000 calories a day. Quite independently we decided to investigate. We interviewed eminent researchers at universities and hospitals throughout Europe and the USA. We delved further into the historical development of Very Low Calorie Diets, checking the results of dozens of medical studies involving thousands of volunteers. Above all, we spoke to scores of the early 'guinea pigs'. Time and time again, these people told the same story. They had lost weight rapidly (some of them for the first time in their lives), they felt well and energetic . . . and, most importantly of all, they had managed to keep their weight down.

Over a period of months, our initial cynicism gave way to an overwhelming conviction that, finally, a real solution to the desperate problem of obesity had been found. There was one major dilemma. This slimming breakthrough was not available to the British public. So we went further. We decided not just to write about The Micro Diet breakthrough but to actually produce it.

Our first step was to approach one of the UK's leading manufacturers of nutritional foodstuffs for hospitals and give them the brief that we wanted to formulate *the best* Very Low Calorie Diet. It would need the ideal balance of protein, carbohydrate, vitamins, minerals and all of the other essential nutrients. The outcome was a 330-calorie a day regime providing complete five-star nutrition. We then arranged for clinical trials to be conducted on this specific formulation at the University of Surrey's Department of Biochemistry. The results were a complete success and impressed even the experienced team of doctors and nutritionists involved.

Within weeks there were hundreds of people on the diet. Many around Guildford where the University of Surrey is situated; others comprised of family, friends and acquaintances. By September 1983, largely through word-of-mouth recommendation, about 1,000 people were on the diet. Their successes and enthusiasm were so noticeable that suddenly thousands of people were clamouring for The Micro Diet. A company trading as Uni-Vite Nutrition was formed to cope with the ever-increasing demand. Through advertising in prestigious

3

medical journals we brought the diet plan to the attention of the health professionals. Many tried the programme for themselves, and soon doctors, health visitors and even sceptical dietitians (when they saw the practical results) began recommending it.

Encouraged by the enthusiastic response we gave up everything and threw ourselves into making the diet available on a larger scale. We felt it would be a success, but never in our wildest dreams did we imagine how big the demand would actually be. Two years later, The Uni-Vite Micro Diet is the number one method of slimming in Britain. At the time of writing there are over 500,000 Micro-Dieters. Our company, Uni-Vite Nutrition, has experienced a whirlwind growth similar to some of the 'high tech' computer giants, and is said by financial experts to be one of the fastest growing companies in the country. The growth of the company has been exciting, of course, and challenging, but what make it so *enjoyable* are the thousands and thousands of letters and phone calls from people who have been so successful in losing weight – many for the first time. And it's not just the weight loss that they are grateful for; many of them comment on a very noticeable improvement in their over-all health.

There have been critics, of course. We knew from the outset that a Very Low Calorie Diet could be controversial *because it breaks new ground and overturns accepted dietary advice.*

We feel that it is all very well to theorise. The real life results, however, really do speak for themselves. Ask the reigning Miss United Kingdom, Mandy Shires, who could not have won the coveted title without losing two stone on The Micro Diet. Ask our first Micro-Dieter of the year, Cornish businessman, John Bray, who shed 6½ stone in as many months. Ask any of the 15,000 Independent Uni-Vite Advisors, people who have been so impressed with their own experience of The Micro Diet that they in turn have decided to help others fashion healthier, trimmer bodies. They provide the vital advice, help, support and

4

encouragement that every slimmer realistically needs to achieve their goal.

In this book we provide the full background to the development of the Very Low Calorie Diet. We give the latest clinical evidence. We tell you what it's like to go on the diet and how to increase your chances of success. We quote some of our slimming stars from all parts of the country – many of whom have already lost 6 or 7 stone, or more, and whose lives have quite literally been transformed. Real people. Real names.

Clearly, the first priority is for you to lose your excess weight. But there is much, much more to The Micro Diet than a highly nutritious, low-calorie product. There is a full and realistic programme for keeping the weight off – *permanently*. And there are dozens of fascinating facts about nutrition included in this book, designed to help you eat and cook in the healthiest way.

We have tried to ensure that this book answers all of the questions you, your doctor or dietitian may want to raise. We have certainly tackled head-on the criticisms that we have heard to date. We make no apology for our enthusiasm. For millions of people, being overweight is a serious, worrying and depressing problem and we are grateful to be involved in a genuine breakthrough that brings a solution within their reach.

Malcolm J. Nicholl

Colin Rose

PART I

THE DIET PLAN

1

DO YOU REALLY NEED
TO LOSE WEIGHT?

Modern western society favours a slim physique. Open the pages of any glossy magazine, watch television 'soaps' or peruse eye-catching advertisements and you'll find that all of the 'beautiful people' obviously living the good life have one thing in common: thin, trim, healthy bodies. No wonder that so many of us seek to emulate the sports stars, or the fashion models. Vanity plays a part. It's only natural that many overweight people want to improve their looks. No wonder that at any time 11½ million people in Britain are following a diet programme.

Concern over one's appearance, however, pales into insignificance as a motivation for losing excess fat, when you begin to consider the health hazards of obesity. Obese people, quite bluntly, are at increased risk of coronary artery disease, high blood pressure, diabetes mellitus and gall bladder disease. At particular risk of developing such conditions are the offspring of people already suffering these ailments. Overweight children are very likely to become obese adults and the British population as a whole is actually continuing to become more overweight in spite of greater efforts at health education.

According to the Royal College of Physicians, the prevalence of overweight increases from 15% in 16–19-year olds to 54% in men and 50% in women aged 60–65 years of age. Taking adults as a whole into account, 39% of men and 32% of women are overweight with 6% of men and 8% of women being classified as obese. (Those at increased risk of early death.) The more overweight you become, the greater the risk. But in its Report on Obesity the Royal College concluded that even mild degrees of overweight are, on a public health basis, important, especially for those people with a family history of cardiovascular disease and diabetes and in people who already have high blood pressure.

What is equally important, however, is that an obsession with being unnaturally thin can also be dangerous. There is nothing wrong with losing weight for cosmetic reasons, but it should never be carried to extremes. For example, there is no evidence that a reasonable degree of overweight is a serious health hazard in people over the age of 40, unless they have an associated disorder. Moreover, it is a biological fact that women tend to store fat in their thighs and buttocks. The actual size of the fat cells are larger in the thigh area of women than in their abdominal area, and this fat is inevitably more difficult to mobilise than in other parts of the body. You should not diet excessively to try to change the natural distribution of fat that evolution has ordained.

Whilst women tend to store fat in their thighs and buttocks, men tend to store fat in their abdomens. In a recent study reported by Professor Bjorntorp of Gothenburg, Sweden, it has become clear that male abdominal obesity – the archetypical 'beer gut' or 'pot belly' – substantially increases the risk of a stroke or heart disease. This risk starts when the waist measures more than the hips.

In other words, you are right to want to ensure you are not overweight, but the risks of obesity vary considerably with age and sex.

Having made these points it is easy to understand why so many people are always seeking *the solution*. Let's be honest. For the most part traditional dietary advice has failed. Less than 10% of people who actually manage to lose their excess weight are able to keep it off in the long term. The 'yo-yo' syndrome (of losing weight and regaining it) is borne out by the depressing statistic that the average slimmer embarks on 14 different diets during the course of her lifetime!

We know, through a survey conducted for us, that 95%

10

of Micro-Dieters have dieted before and failed. All too frequently, they reveal a lifetime on a slimming treadmill. We've attended countless meetings where many depressed overweight women (and men) will state 'I've tried *everything*' – and then back it up with a list of failures . . . calorie counting, high-protein diets, high-carbohydrate diets, or low-carbohydrate diets, high-fibre diets, the grapefruit diet, egg diets, the beer drinker's diet – the list is endless.

They will talk about attending weekly slimming clubs for months without losing weight or they will have been to the doctor for diuretics or injections. Some will have resorted to acupuncture, hypnosis or total starvation. We have even heard of extreme cases where women have been into hospital for surgery – gastroplasty or stomach stapling – while others have had their jaws wired. Maybe friends will have told them to simply cut down, or, more crudely, just keep their mouths shut. It's not as easy as that. If it were there would not be the millions of unhappy, overweight people in the country today.

Now however, the latest studies show just why the traditional 1,000-calorie diets have failed.

The answer lies in the body's metabolic rate. This is the rate at which the calories in food are converted to energy. We now know that many more people than previously suspected have an abnormally low metabolic rate. The lady who claims she only has to 'look at a chocolate to gain a pound', may not be so far from the truth after all! She may well have a low metabolic rate and therefore will not burn calories as efficiently as her slim friend.

The official UK government statistics assess the average metabolic rate for a man at 2,800 calories a day and a woman at 2,100 calories a day. That's the number of calories that can be consumed whilst stabilising their weight. But, by definition, an average is made up of women who have a higher metabolic rate – and millions who have a lower metabolic rate. Indeed, Dr Denis Craddock, an authority on slimming, says, 'Some women will in fact gain weight on a routine such as that of Weight

Watchers where they are encouraged to eat about 1,500 calories a day'.

After naturally slim people have eaten, their body increases the amount of heat it produces. This is called 'the thermic response to food'. If they overeat, this extra heat automatically burns off the unwanted calories. Unfortunately, this natural regulator seems to function poorly in some overweight people. Instead of automatically burning off these unwanted calories, they tend to be stored as fat. Furthermore, the metabolic rate of fat people does not increase as much in response to cold as does that of thinner people. Now, the general assumption is that a woman with a below normal metabolism of, say, 1,700 calories a day, and who is on a 1,000-calorie diet, will have a 'calorie deficit' of 700 calories. This calorie deficit will cause her to lose weight as the missing 700 calories are burned from unwanted body fat.

The principle is correct, the figure is wrong. The fact that is too often overlooked is that as soon as one goes on a diet the body, sensing a reduction in calories, reacts defensively by metabolising the food it is receiving more efficiently. The result is that the metabolic rate drops by an average of about 15%. This reduction in metabolic rate occurs on any calorie restricted diet – whether conventional or Very Low Calorie.

The result is that a metabolic rate of 1,700 calories a day will, in fact, drop to about 1,450 calories. So the true deficit is only 450 calories if the woman stays on a 1,000-calorie diet. Since there are 3,500 calories in 1 lb. of human fat, the rate at which fat will be lost is only 2 oz. a day or about 1 lb. every seven days. Even allowing for the accompanying water loss this is discouragingly slow. All too often the dieter considers the results not worth the effort and gives up. If she takes the alternative route, which is to drastically cut her food intake below the 1,000 calorie level, then it is literally impossible to obtain adequate nutrition using conventional solid food. So now she will feel tired and unwell – and again give up. *This vicious circle is the central reason why conventional diets have failed.*

12

Case history

Name: Bernadette Thomas
Home town: Bristol
Weight loss: 4 st. 4 lb.

As soon as she started The Micro Diet, Bernadette Thomas knew it was going to work. She was so confident, in fact, that although she was a size 22 she ordered a size 14 dress to wear to a friend's wedding just seven months away.

Bernadette, a Bristol housewife, did it with weeks to spare. From 14 st. 10 lb. with hips of more than 50 inches, she slimmed to 10 st. 6 lb. with 39½-inch hips.

'I was a porker all my life,' says Bernadette, 27. 'The last time my weight was as low as it is now was when I was 10 years old. I was a 'professional' dieter until I tried The Micro Diet and realised immediately that it was different from everything else I'd tried. After the first few days I wasn't hungry at all and I began to feel so good. I used to be tired and lethargic all the time. Now I'm brimming with energy.'

Adds mother-of-three Bernadette, 'Quite honestly I was so ashamed of myself I used to hide behind the front door whenever I had to open it. Yet, the other day I got my first-ever wolf whistle. Just imagine!'

So why should The Micro Diet succeed when all else has failed? Why should you embark on yet another diet? Why should you even *read* any more of yet another diet book?

Because the diet really does work. Micro-Dieters have proven for themselves the validity of our claims. They see the fat disappearing at such a dramatic rate that they have the incentive to continue until they reach their goal. In a University of Surrey survey of Micro-Dieters a staggering 94% declared that it was easier to lose weight with our plan than previous methods they had tried.

13

Because The Micro Diet already has an enviable track record. More than 500,000 slimmers in just two years; thousands and thousands of delighted dieters who are now proudly just a shadow of their former selves; and not one serious health problem attributable to the diet.

Because they are provided with the crucial support and encouragement of an Independent Uni-Vite Advisor, someone who has succeeded with the diet herself and can, therefore, speak from personal experience. In the survey some 77% of the respondents described the role of the Advisor as 'important' in their success.

Because The Micro Diet plan will help you stay slim. Again, the figures speak for themselves. An amazing 86% found it 'easy' or 'easier' to maintain their target weight.

How much do you need to lose?

Before commencing the diet you must have a clear idea of your goal. It is not sufficient to say 'I want to get rid of a few stone' or 'I'll just see how it goes'. A target is essential.

You know that you are labouring under excess fat – but how much? Quite probably you've checked your situation before with one of the 'weight for height' charts published by the life insurance companies. A more accurate guideline can be ascertained with a method most *informed* experts are now using – the Body Mass Index or BMI. To discover your BMI you take your weight in kilos and divide it by your height in metres squared, i.e.

$$\frac{\text{Weight Kilos}}{\text{Height Metres}^2}$$

As most of us are not mathematicians, we have provided a table to let you check your own BMI – although this will not be as accurate as doing the calculation yourself. The point to note is that you are medically obese if your BMI is 30 or over – and you should do something about it!

To calculate your Body Mass Index

Convert your weight from stones into pounds (1 stone = 14 pounds) and multiply by 0.454 to obtain weight in kilograms. Then, with reference to the height chart provided on page 16, divide this figure by your height in metres squared. The resulting number is your Body Mass Index.

Example
Your weight is 10 st. 2 lb., or 142 lb.
In kilograms: $142 \times 0.454 = 64.5$ kg.
Your height is 5′ 3″, or in metres squared is 2.56.
Therefore your Body Mass Index is $\frac{64.5}{2.56} = 25.2$

Desirable Body Mass Index
The desirable Body Mass Index for medium-frame men regardless of height is 22, but can range from 21.9 to 22.4. For medium-frame women the desirable Index is 21.5 but can range from 21.3 to 22.1.

The formula can be used in reverse. If you know your height and your desirable Body Mass Index, you can obtain your ideal weight by multiplying the ideal Body Mass Index by your height in metres squared.

Your commitment

This book will tell you exactly how to achieve your goal of slimming to your ideal weight. But it cannot do it for you. You must make a commitment! You must want wholeheartedly to win the battle over your weight problem as much as the Olympic athlete wants the gold medal.

The stories of our triumphant 'losers' should motivate you. People like Anne Platt of Yorkshire who got rid of more than five stone in five months and now, at 10 st. 7 lb., 'feels like a different person'; Maureen Harris of Bournemouth, who is thrilled because after losing 8½ stone she can cut her own toenails; Monica Ogden of Sheffield, 4½ stone lighter, who is 'no longer ashamed' of

IDEAL WEIGHT RANGE

HEIGHT			WOMEN (Medium Frame)		MEN (Medium Frame)	
Metric (Metres)	Imperial (Ft., in.)	Height in m²	Metric	Imperial	Metric	Imperial
1.425m	4ft. 8in.	2.03m²	43.2–44.9kg	6st. 11lb. – 7st. 1lb.		
1.450m	4ft. 9in.	2.10m²	44.7–46.4kg	7st. 0lb. – 7st. 4lb.		
1.475m	4ft. 10in.	2.18m²	46.4–48.2kg	7st. 4lb. – 7st. 8lb.		
1.500m	4ft. 11in.	2.25m²	47.9–49.7kg	7st. 7lb. – 7st. 11lb.		
1.525m	5ft. 0in.	2.33m²	49.6–51.5kg	7st. 11lb. – 8st. 1lb.		
1.550m	5ft. 1in.	2.40m²	51.1–53.0kg	8st. 0lb. – 8st. 5lb.	52.6–53.8kg	8st. 4lb. – 8st. 6lb.
1.575m	5ft. 2in.	2.48m²	52.8–54.8kg	8st. 4lb. – 8st. 9lb.	54.3–55.5kg	8st. 7lb. – 8st. 10lb.
1.600m	5ft. 3in.	2.56m²	54.5–56.6kg	8st. 8lb. – 8st. 13lb.	56.1–57.3kg	8st. 11lb. – 9st. 0lb.
1.625m	5ft. 4in.	2.64m²	56.2–58.3kg	8st–12lb. – 9st. 2lb.	57.8–59.1kg	9st. 1lb. – 9st. 4lb.
1.650m	5ft. 5in.	2.72m²	57.9–60.1kg	9st. 1lb. – 9st. 6lb.	59.6–60.9kg	9st. 5lb. – 9st. 8lb.
1.675m	5ft. 6in.	2.81m²	59.8–62.1kg	9st. 6lb. – 9st. 11lb.	61.5–62.9kg	9st. 9lb. – 9st. 12lb.
1.700m	5ft. 7in.	2.89m²	61.6–63.9kg	9st. 10lb. – 10st. 1lb.	63.3–64.7kg	9st. 13lb. – 10st. 2lb.
1.725m	5ft. 8in.	2.98m²	63.5–65.9kg	10st. 0lb. – 10st. 5lb.	65.3–66.7kg	10st. 4lb. – 10st. 7lb.
1.750m	5ft. 9in.	3.06m²	65.2–67.6kg	10st. 3lb. – 10st. 9lb.	67.0–68.5kg	10st. 7lb. – 10st. 11lb.
1.775m	5ft. 10in.	3.15m²	67.1–69.6kg	10st. 8lb. – 10st. 13lb.	69.0–70.6kg	10st. 12lb. – 11st. 1lb.
1.800m	5ft. 11in.	3.24m²	69.0–71.6kg	10st. 12lb. – 11st. 4lb.	71.0–72.6kg	11st. 2lb. – 11st. 6lb.
1.825m	6ft. 0in.	3.33m²			72.9–74.6kg	11st. 6lb. – 11st. 10lb.
1.850m	6ft. 1in.	3.42m²			74.9–76.6kg	11st. 11lb. – 12st. 1lb.
1.875m	6ft. 2in.	3.52m²			77.1–78.8kg	12st. 2lb. – 12st. 5lb.
1.900m	6ft. 3in.	3.61m²			79.1–80.9kg	12st. 6lb. – 12st. 10lb.

the way she looks; 22-year-old Joanne Butler, of London, who lost 4 stone and gained her first pair of jeans; and polio victim Janet Hallpatch of Southampton whose specially reinforced callipers broke under her 18½-stone frame, who has melted away 5½ of her excess stone in seven months.

As part of The Micro Diet programme you will also have an Advisor to be your 'helping hand'. The rest is up to you.

Whatever the amount you need to lose you have to acknowledge the fact. You then have your target. You know that being obese is associated with severe health problems and you probably don't care for the way you look.

Answer 'yes' to the following statements before proceeding further.

MY COMMITMENT

I am going to succeed with the Micro Diet because

I am personally too overweight for my own good and I know it is jeopardising my health and happiness.   Yes/No

I really want to look younger and more attractive. Yes/No

I would be more responsible to my family if I lost weight and improved my health.   Yes/No

I want to feel more energetic and become more active.

Yes/No

I am NOT just 'giving it a try', I am making a serious effort.   Yes/No

I know it will work – if I work with it.   Yes/No

2

THE BREAKTHROUGH

The Very Low Calorie Diet is not an overnight success story. Dedicated scientific research stretching back more than 50 years, lies behind the programme now sweeping the country.

Scientific attention has, however, in the last few years become focused more clearly on VLCDs as the real solution to obesity. There is now more clinical evidence – published and unpublished – to support a VLCD regime than any other method available today, and more studies continue to be conducted around the world. Consistently, they show that Very Low Calorie Diets can be used effectively and safely – even for those people who have failed on traditional 1,000-calorie programmes. For many scientists are convinced that there are more people than originally suspected whose metabolic rate is so low that they will never lose weight on a conventional diet. For them, old-style diet advice is a cruel deception.

Strangely, it was as long ago as the 1930s that researchers first seriously considered very low calorie plans. A group of American doctors devised 400–600-calorie a day diets – using conventional food, of course. As a result the diets were nutritionally deficient (in those days, in fact, some vitamins and minerals had not even been discovered). Nevertheless, the results were successful. Over 300 patients monitored by researchers Strang, McClugage and Evans at the Western Pennsylvania Hospital in Pittsburgh, lost an average of 22 pounds over eight weeks with no ill effects. In spite of their triumphs, they did not pursue their studies further and it was to be years before anyone else took up the research.

The next stage, actually, was a backward one, when complete starvation went through a phase of popularity in the 1950s. It is hard to comprehend why such 'zero calorie–zero nutrition' programmes were pursued. Not surprisingly, spectacular weight losses were achieved but the body's vital organs were placed at serious risk and, in fact, such diets led to deaths . . . even with hospital patients under constant medical supervision. Then, very low-calorie high-protein regimes were explored, primarily in the United States and France. Tragically, this pioneering work led to the marketing of a 'liquid protein' diet in the US. These diets contained collagen, a low-quality protein lacking certain essential amino acids; they contained no carbohydrate; and were also deficient in selenium and electrolytes – highly necessary for the heart to function properly. A large number of deaths were attributed to the 'liquid protein' diet owing to heart problems and the diet, quite rightly, was banned. The sad episode cast an unjustified cloud over the development of Very Low Calorie Diets.

Some tenacious researchers, however, would not give up. Quietly, on both sides of the Atlantic, they were studying the benefits of formulations that included *all* of the essential nutrients and *a balance* of protein, carbohydrate and fat. In the United States, doctors at the Mount Sinai Hospital in Cleveland, and Harvard Medical School, Boston, conducted studies with protein as the dominant food component. In Europe, there was much research using carbohydrate as the primary source. Studies were held at the University of Cambridge and at other hospitals in Dublin, Naples, Amsterdam, Rotterdam, Copenhagen and Gothenburg.

Time and again these independent researchers found their patients losing weight rapidly . . . just as quickly as they would on a dangerous starvation plan but without the serious side effects. On the contrary, significant health improvements were noted:

  * Cholesterol and triglyceride levels dropped for those patients with high levels.

* Hypertensive patients noticed a dramatic drop in blood pressure.
* Diabetic patients, too, recorded beneficial lowering of blood glucose.

There have now been dozens of clinical trials on VLCDs involving more than 15,000 patients under rigorous medical supervision. The most comprehensive and independent assessment of the effectiveness and safety of VLCDs was reported recently by one of the world's foremost medical journals, *The Annals of Internal Medicine*, which is published by the American College of Physicians.

Written by a team from the University of Pennsylvania, Dr Thomas Wadden, Dr Albert Stunkard and Dr Kelly Brownell, all major researchers in the field of obesity, it reported that Very Low Calorie Diets safely produce average weight losses of 15–22 pounds in a month and at least 44 pounds over 12 weeks.

Their conclusions: 'As contrasted to the earlier "liquid protein" diets that were associated with at least 60 deaths, VLCDs of high-quality protein appear safe when limited to 3 months or less under careful medical supervision'. The safety evidence, they stated, was of round-the-clock monitoring of heart action and the fact that no diet-related fatalities had been reported in over 10,000 cases. These cases, it should be emphasised, were subjects who specifically took part in clinical trials, whereas of course, there are now *millions* of members of the public worldwide who have used VLCDs successfully and safely.

Effectiveness

Weight losses on a VLCD are 'far greater' than for other non-surgical treatments, as conventional treatments for obesity, including behaviour modification, diet and anorectic drugs, produce average losses of less than 15 lb., said the American researchers. They added, 'Only 10% of patients treated with conventional therapies *ever* achieve 20 kg (44 lb.), the *average* weight loss for 12 weeks on a VLCD.'

Safety

Another leading American researcher, Dr Victor Vertes, calculates the expected fatality rate for obese people as 4 in 1,000. So in the survey of 10,000 people some 40 fatalities might have been expected – yet there were none. The effect of VLCDs, therefore, was to increase health and safety. Comparing VLCDs with the use of diuretics, the Pennsylvania doctors suggested VLCDs 'may be safer than diuretic agents in the treatment of hypertension in the obese'.

The survey authors then turned their attention to cardiac performance – since, with the grossly inadequate liquid protein diets, heart irregularities were found to be the principle health hazard. Their conclusion was again very clear. *'Cardiac performance is not adversely affected by very low calorie diets of high-quality protein; in fact it may actually be improved.'*

The authors do make the point that in the absence of long-term monitoring, they 'would suggest limiting VLCDs to periods not to exceed 12 weeks'. Since an average weight loss of over three stone is to be expected in this period, this is hardly a major restriction.

The researchers further stress (and we strongly concur) that careful medical supervision is necessary, because there are some contra-indications to the use of VLCDs – kidney disease, a recent heart attack, and pregnancy, for example.

Medical benefits

Apart from the obvious benefit of a VLCD – that of producing a realistically fast and therefore motivating weight loss – Doctors Wadden, Stunkard and Brownell concluded that there were significant medical benefits.

Reduction in blood pressure
They commented, 'There are many reports of large reduction in systolic and diastolic blood pressure'. For

instance in 12 weeks studies, one group of researchers noted 'a decline in mean arterial pressure from 102mm Hg to 84.5mm Hg'. Another reported 'a decline from 111mm Hg to 95mm Hg.'

Reduction in serum cholesterol
'Significant decreases in serum total cholesterol of 20% to 25%' were noted in several studies.

Improvement in Diabetics
The American doctors stated, 'Several reports have shown the effectiveness of VLCDs in the short-term control of Type II diabetes'. Researchers, they said, reported 'discontinuing insulin within one week in seven patients needing 30 to 100 units' and 'normal glucose levels after only four days of dieting'. (Under no circumstances should a diabetic patient use the diet without medical supervision.)

Psychological
'Dieting may be accompanied by a number of untoward emotional responses. Researchers using VLCDs, however, have reported few such responses,' they said.

Side effects
'Side effects of VLCDs are generally mild and easily managed. Postural hypotension (dizziness) is common, but is corrected by plentiful intake of water'. (The incidence 'fewer than 10%'.) Patients had been able to either maintain their normal activity level while dieting or actually increase it, said the researchers.

Follow up care
Turning their attention to long-term weight maintenance they observed, 'Follow up care is essential to the maintenance of weight loss, and may include further nutrition education, training in behavioural methods of diet control and increased physical activity. Although group treatment is the most economical approach, some

researchers believe individual counselling is more effective'.

The future

The eminent researchers concluded: 'Large rapid weight losses and reductions in risk factors make the use of very low calorie diets attractive . . . Attention must be directed to the problem of maintenance of weight losses'.

'A comprehensive programme combining VLCDs (to achieve a large initial weight loss) with nutrition education, exercise, training and behaviour modification would appear to be the next step.'

THIS CONCLUSION, THEN, FROM THE MOST COMPREHENSIVE *INDEPENDENT* REPORT ON VLCD'S AND BASED ON A FULL SURVEY OF THE LITERATURE AND MAIN MEDICAL TRIALS, EXACTLY DESCRIBES THE MICRO DIET PROGRAMME.

The Micro Diet plan – which will be fully detailed in this book – incorporates:
1. a proven effective VLCD.
2. important information on nutrition.
3. advice on changing cooking and eating habits to permanently reduce calorie intake, plus
4. the personal advice, encouragement and support of the National Advisor Service.

Case history

Name: Ruth Fitzpatrick
Home town: Doncaster
Weight loss: 3 st. 7 lb.

During 27 years as a nurse caring for other people, Ruth Fitzpatrick was fighting her own personal battle against ill health and overweight.

She saw herself as a 'fat little barrel' who made excuses for avoiding social occasions.

She tried high-protein diets, high-fibre diets, egg diets, lemon juice and lettuce leaf diets and even hypnotism. At 5 feet tall and 12 st. 4 lb. she needed to slim, not just for appearance's sake but because she has only one kidney and her overweight condition was damaging her health.

Three and a half stone later, Ruth of Doncaster, Yorks, says: 'I look and feel 10 years younger. My kidney function has improved and I don't need to take any tablets. It's marvellous.'

3

THE MICRO DIET:
WHAT IS IN IT AND WHY

The Micro Diet is a simple regime involving 3 or 4 very low-calorie, but highly nutritious, drinks a day. They come in various flavours and are remarkably satisfying. Each 'meal' has just 110 calories and at that level of calorie intake, you *must* lose weight. There is no doubt that The Micro Diet works. The clinical evidence and public experience – which we will describe later – is now very convincing.

But let's examine just what makes The Micro Diet so special. Three Micro Diet meals a day serve carefully measured amounts of all the nutrients necessary for a healthy body. It is absolutely no use consuming megadoses of one nutrient only to be deficient in another, equally important, one. After all, your body is more complex than the most sophisticated computer and requires an army of more than 50 essential nutrients often inter-acting to keep it functioning. These nutrients have to (a) furnish the fuel, (b) build and maintain body tissues, and (c) regulate body processes.

Here is what you obtain in one day's supply of The Micro Diet. (A more detailed breakdown of the nutritional components of The Micro Diet can be found in Appendix A at the back of the book.)

42 grams of Protein
Protein provides the 22 different amino acids that build our bodies and tissues. Of these, eight are called 'essential' (nine for infants) because the body cannot make them: they have to come from the food we eat. Every single body cell contains protein: the skin, teeth

25

and nails, hair and bones. As these body proteins are continuously broken down, and some protein is lost, the body's protein stores have to be constantly replenished.

If you read the tables produced by most governments you will find some variation in the average amount of protein recommended. The US government recommends an average of 56 grams for men and 44 grams for women. That assumes a mixed diet of high- and low-grade protein and is increased by 30 per cent over the minimum levels to account for individual variations. The World Health Organisation recommends 37 grams of protein daily. The UK government recommends higher figures, averaging 65 grams per day for men and 54 grams for women. These recommendations, of course, also assume that the average diet includes a mixture of high- and low-grade protein and is for people on a weight maintenance programme.

Clinical trials have clearly shown that the 42 grams of pure high-grade protein in three servings of the Micro Diet – for women – and the 56 grams in four Micro Diet servings (or 59 grams in three servings plus 1½ ounces of skimmed milk) – for men – is absolutely sufficient.

35 grams of Carbohydrate

A primary function of digestible carbohydrate is to serve as a major source of energy for the body.

All of the nutrients work together to promote a healthy body and this is particularly true of carbohydrate and protein. Carbohydrate operates hand in glove with protein to make the action of the protein more efficient. If there were not enough carbohydrate in the diet, the body would break down protein to provide carbohydrate for the brain to use, 'stealing' protein from its main purpose of repairing tissues and promoting growth. Digestible carbohydrates also promote normal fat metabolism, help prevent loss of sodium and involuntary dehydration.

3 grams of Fat

Fat in the diet is necessary to provide the essential fatty acids but it does 'cost' nine calories per gram or 252 calories per ounce, so we need enough, but not too much.

Without fat, vitamins A, D, E and K could not be absorbed into our bodies.

1500 mg of Sodium, 2010 mg of Potassium, 1800 mg of Chloride

These three electrolytes work together to nourish body cells. In balanced proportions they are essential for muscle and nerve activity. They also help acid balance of body fluids. A deficiency can cause tiredness and irregular heart beats. Sodium chloride is the chemical name given to common salt, so foods rich in this condiment – such as processed and preserved products – are also high in sodium and chloride. Potassium is present in most common foods in moderate amounts. Fruit, vegetables and instant coffee are rich sources.

It is worth noting, however, too much sodium may cause water retention and hypertension. Some people are particularly sensitive to excessive salt in their diet. As The Micro Diet has relatively low salt content it can be particularly beneficial to those people.

900 mg of Calcium, 800 mg of Phosphorus

Calcium and Phosphorus build strong bones and teeth. So they are particularly important for expectant mothers and babies and children. These nutrients need the help of Vitamin D to be effective. The most valuable sources of calcium are milk and cheese. However, pulses and other vegetables also contribute calcium to the diet. In general, rich food sources of calcium are also rich in phosphorus.

350 mg of Magnesium

Magnesium is essential for all living cells for the functioning of some of the enzymes involved in energy utilisation. It helps muscles keep working. Most natural foods contain useful amounts of magnesium; cereals and vegetables make particularly valuable contributions.

20 mg of Iron

Iron keeps your blood healthy! It forms part of the red pigments of blood, which carries oxygen from your lungs to every part of your body and takes the waste product, carbon dioxide, back to your lungs. Sources of iron are liver, kidney (and black pudding).

20 mg of Zinc

This trace element is needed for growth, wound healing, skin health and resistance to infection. Good dietary sources in daily use are meats, legumes and whole grains.

2 mg of Copper

Copper is an essential trace element which forms part of many enzyme systems. Its metabolism in the body is closely related to that of iron. Deficiency causes anaemia. Green vegetables, many species of fish, oysters and liver are all good sources of copper, but most other foods provide only small amounts.

2.9 mg of Manganese

This is a trace element associated with a number of enzymes. Deficiency causes poor growth and bone deformities in animals. The average British diet provides 4.6 mg. a day, half of which comes from tea. Other rich sources are whole cereals, legumes and leafy vegetables.

0.16 mg of Molybdenum

This is a trace element which forms a vital part of several enzyme systems. It may help prevent tooth decay. Among the richest sources of molybdenum are cabbage, carrots, potatoes and broad beans.

150 ug of Iodine

Iodine is vital to the metabolism. It contributes to the hormones thyroxine and triodothyronine which help regulate metabolic rate. Fish is the only rich source of iodine. Fruits, vegetables, cereals and meat provide varying amounts.

Fat soluble vitamins

1.0 mg of Vitamin A

Vitamin A is essential for vision in dim light and for the maintenance of healthy skin, eyes and hair – surface tissue in general. It is found mainly in milk, butter, cheese, egg yolks, liver and some fatty fish. However, carotenes can be converted into Vitamin A in the body and rich sources of these pigments include carrots, leafy vegetables and apricots.

11 ug of Vitamin D

This vitamin is required for strong teeth and bones. It maintains the level of calcium and phosphorus in the blood. Fish liver oils are by far the richest dietary source but this vitamin can also be formed in the body by sunlight reacting in the skin.

10 mg of Vitamin E

Despite widespread publicity, Vitamin E may not be essential for man! It is believed to serve a function in keeping blood cells healthy and it does counteract rancidity in fats. The richest sources are vegetable oils and, therefore, margarine and shortening also provide considerable amounts.

70 ug of Vitamin K

Vitamin K is necessary for the normal clotting of blood. The best sources are fresh leafy vegetables.

Water soluble vitamins

70 mg of Vitamin C

Necessary for healthy connective tissue, teeth, gums and bones, Vitamin C also builds strong body cells and blood vessels. Fresh fruit and green leafy vegetables are rich sources of this vitamin. Potatoes are not a particularly good source but as large amounts may be eaten they can be the major provider of Vitamin C.

2 mg of Thiamin, Vitamin B1

This is required for the steady and continuous release of energy from carbohydrates. A deficiency of this vitamin produces beri-beri. The best sources are brewers yeast, marmite and bran.

2 mg of Riboflavin, Vitamin B2

Riboflavin is necessary for healthy skin, building and maintaining body tissues, concerned with the sensitivity of the eyes to light and required for the releasing of energy from food. It is found in significant amounts in liver, milk, eggs and green vegetables but, in contrast to other B vitamins, it is relatively lacking in cereal grains.

3 mg of Pyridoxine, Vitamin B6

This is involved in the metabolism of amino acids. It is necessary for the formation of haemoglobin and the proper functioning of the nervous system. Good sources include liver, whole grain cereals, peanuts and bananas, but most foods are moderate sources.

19 mg of Niacin

This is required to convert food to energy, aid the nervous system, and to maintain a healthy skin. Humans do not rely totally on dietary intake of this vitamin as it may also be synthesised from tryptophan, one of the essential amino acids.

7 mg of Pantothenic Acid

This is necessary for the release of energy from fat and carbohydrate. It is also required for tissue growth. The richest sources of Pantothenic Acid include liver, kidney, yeast, bran and egg yolk.

0.4 mg of Folic Acid

In conjunction with B12, this is essential for healthy blood formation and is important in tissues where cells are dividing rapidly, e.g. pregnancy. It can be deficient in many diets. Found in liver, kidney, spinach and broccoli tops.

0.2 mg of Biotin

This is essential for the metabolism of fat. The richest sources are liver, kidney and yeast extract but many species of bacteria can make or retain biotin, so humans can probably obtain all they need from micro-organisms in food and in the gut.

5 ug of Vitamin B12

Working with Folic Acid, this is essential for healthy blood formation and the nervous system. It is only found in foods of animal origin.

Together, these provide the nutrients your body needs, thus avoiding the dangerous deficiencies associated with conventional severe diets or, even worse, fasting. If you find it difficult to visualise just how much nutrition is concentrated into the 330 calories of The Micro Diet, the next table certainly brings it into perspective.

The Micro Diet gives a slimmer a complete day's nutrition – in the same number of calories as in one small bar of chocolate! In fact, as a source of protein and basic nutrition, it is proportionately cheaper than the chocolate bar!

A COMPARISON OF THREE FOODS
ALL THREE CONTAIN 330 CALORIES!

		3 Servings Uni-Vite Micro Diet(100g)	One Yorkie Bar i.e. 2.1 oz. choc.	3½ oz. of boiled sweets (100g)
Calories		330	330	330
Protein	g	42	5	trace
Carbohydrate	g	35	37	87
Fat	g	3	19	trace
Calcium	mg	900	137	5
Iron	mg	20	1	0.4
Potassium	mg	2010	262	8
Sodium	mg	1500	75	25
Magnesium	mg	350	34	2
Phosphorus	mg	800	150	12
Chloride	mg	1800	168	68
Copper	mg	2	trace	trace
Zinc	mg	20	0.1	0
Manganese	mg	3	?	?
Iodine	mcg	150	?	?
Molybdenum	mcg	160	?	?
Selenium	mcg	60	?	?
Chromium	mcg	60	?	?

VITAMIN

A	mg	1	4.2	0
Folic Acid	mcg	400	6.2	0
Biotin	mcg	200	1.9	0
Pantothenic Acid	mg	7	0.37	0
Thiamin	mg	2	0.06	0
E	mg	10	0.3	0
Niacin	mg	19	0.1	0
Riboflavin	mg	2	0.14	0
B6	mg	3	trace	0
B12	mcg	5	trace	0
C	mg	70	0	0
D	mcg	11	trace	0
K	mcg	70	?	?
Choline	mg	450	?	?
Inositol	mg	120	?	?

4

GETTING STARTED

Take a deep breath – and start on the path to a trimmer body. Just imagine what it will be like to have lost those extra stones, to be lighter on your feet, to be able to wear stylish clothes, to feel and be healthier. It's worth the effort!

Consult your doctor

Your first step, of course, as with any diet, is to visit your G.P. so that he can establish your initial state of health and the advisability of a Very Low Calorie Diet for you personally. Some doctors will not be familiar with VLCDs, so we have provided a short description of The Micro Diet for your G.P. Take this book with you and show your G.P. Appendix B on page 156.

Take a picture

Once you have the 'all clear', and even before your first Micro Diet meal, take a picture of yourself. Most overweight people tend to shy away from cameras but once you've slimmed down you'll want a photograph to proudly prove your achievement and as a constant reminder not to slip back.

Weigh in

Accurately weigh yourself and make sure that throughout your diet plan you weigh yourself at the same time every day wearing the same clothes or none at all.

First thing in the morning is usually a good idea. Work out
how much weight you need to lose (go back to the BMI
chart in Chapter 1).

Morale-booster

Find a way of recording your progress. Some slimmers
like to fill a box with heavy objects – books or stones for
instance – to represent that excess weight. As the pounds
disappear they remove the corresponding weight in
objects. It's wonderfully encouraging to find yourself
physically 'throwing away the fat' – representing less and
less strain on your heart and lungs.

If this is too time-consuming or the box takes up too much
space, you could set two glass jars near the bathroom scales.
Place marbles into one jar – each marble counting as one of
your unwanted pounds – and transfer the marbles according
to your weight loss. It will be a positive morale-booster!

Dieting made easy

'Flexibility' and 'simplicity' are the key words of The
Micro Diet programme.

Flexibility means the ability to adapt the basic programme to suit your own individual lifestyle.

We don't feel it is at all appropriate to lay down rigid
guidelines and insist that you obey them. We don't see
the point in anyone becoming a martyr to a diet regime
and we certainly don't want you to suffer excruciating
pangs of guilt because you 'sneaked' a chocolate biscuit.
After all, as our plans are so low in calories, *a few* extra
calories are not going to be as disastrous as a few extra
would be when added to a traditional 1,000-calorie plan.
That's why we like to think of The Micro Diet as the
benevolent diet.

Simplicity means that The Micro Diet takes the guesswork
out of slimming. Its perfect nutritional content in so few
calories makes it a sophisticated diet; yet following the
programme itself couldn't be easier.

You don't have to count calories or weigh foods. You
don't have to search the supermarkets for exotic fruits and
vegetables. You don't have to spend hours in the kitchen.
You don't have to spend a fortune to attend a weekly
slimming meeting, or pay even when you don't attend.

With The Micro Diet you know *exactly* how many
calories you are consuming. You know *exactly* the fine
balance of nutrients being fed to your body. With
traditional diets, you're tempted every step of the way –
shopping, preparing the food and cooking the meal. It is
so easy to allow yourself a 'small' extra portion or 'forget
yourself' and just have a 'little taste'. Before long your
1,000-calorie plan has had several hundred extra un-
counted calories added to it. The Micro Diet removes the
temptation and the evidence is that you probably won't be
hungry, in any case.

The Micro Diet

As The Micro Diet is food in powdered form it can
provide all of your nutritional needs without the calories,
forming what a top nutritionist at the University of
Heidelberg has called 'the perfect food'.

35

We totally understand that when you're used to consuming large quantities of food, it's hard to imagine how you could be satisfied by a liquid regime. The truth, as confirmed by thousands of Micro-Dieters, is that the drinks and soups, in eight flavours, are immensely filling. The slimmer can happily replace meals at any time of the day because they are available in sweets and savouries: Chocolate, Vanilla, Strawberry, Butterscotch, Banana, Coffee, Beef soup and Chicken and Herb soup.

All you have to do is take one sachet of the powder, mix it with half a pint of cold or hot water (not boiling) and you have an appetising, nourishing meal. You know that you are consuming exactly 110 calories and that you are obtaining one-third of the recommended daily amounts of protein, vitamins, minerals, trace elements and electrolytes. Vitamin and mineral tablets should not be taken in addition. The unique carob-coated Micro Meal, a high-fibre, high-protein food bar – just 250 calories – can also be effectively used as part of a Uni-Vite weight loss plan to add variety and provide something to chew. There are several Uni-Vite plans, ranging from the minimum of 330 calories a day to 750 calories a day.

And there are many options for the way in which you adapt the diet plan to suit your own lifestyle. For instance, if you are carrying several extra stone you could follow the 'sole source' plan Mondays to Fridays and eat 'normally' at the weekends – or at least have your traditional Sunday lunch. Alternatively, you could use The Micro Diet meals on a 'one day on – one day off' basis. Your doctor will be able to guide you.

Often, Micro-Dieters find that it is best to set themselves a short-term target – an initial five days of 'sole source'. The weight loss during that time can be so exciting that the slimmer has no hesitation in continuing with the plan. And, after a lifetime of gaining weight, just five days serious dieting is no great sacrifice, and many people report losses of over 1 lb. a day straight away.

Case history

Name: Peter Kelly
Home town: Liverpool
Weight loss: 4 st. 7 lb.

Peter Kelly had a shock when he went to the doctor with a knee injury: the doctor was more interested in his excess fat and ordered him to lose weight.

Twenty-one-stone Peter from Hale, Liverpool, took the advice seriously, although he had tried to lose weight before and failed. When he heard about The Micro Diet he was openly sceptical but realised he had nothing to lose – except several stone. The first days on The Micro Diet left him feeling off-colour but, encouraged by his wife, Kay, he persevered.

Peter went on to drop 4½ stone in three months while Kay shed two stone to reach her target weight. Says Peter: 'My doctor was delighted with my success and, I must confess, I actually enjoyed dieting. I found most of the Uni-Vite flavours quite tasty and satisfying even though I ate nothing else for three weeks at a time. I included a meal during the fourth week but found it easy to go back on the sole source plan.'

The Micro Diet options

Variety is the spice of life.

Don't make the mistake of thinking that a liquid-only plan must be boring or like 'taking medicine'. Far from it! The Micro Diet programme has been designed to satisfy your taste buds any hour of the day. And there are many ways of turning your Micro Diet meal into a real treat, hot or cold, ideally replacing breakfast, lunch and dinner.

How to mix

A sachet of The Micro Diet should always be added to water (not the other way round). It is not necessary to have expensive equipment to mix a smooth, creamy drink. The formula can be easily mixed with a variety of implements. Top of the range is obviously a liquidiser which ensures a smooth consistency – but also means washing up. A hand blender is just as effective and easier to clean (but put the blender into the mixture before turning on – otherwise your ceiling might receive the benefit). If you don't have access to such gadgets, there are various plastic shakers on the market which, with a little vigorous shaking, will do the job. Another word of caution: using hot water or carbonated beverages can literally have an explosive effect. A wire spring whisk with a bowl or even a clean screw-top jar (a coffee jar, for instance) can also be used to mix the formula. Never use boiling water as this can destroy some of the nutrients, and consume the meal immediately after preparing so that no nutrients are lost.

Presentation

Sometimes we do 'eat with our eyes'. So why not serve up your Chicken and Herb or Beef soup in a soup bowl, garnished according to your preference and sit down at the dinner table with the rest of the family? Present yourself with a Chocolate, Strawberry or Vanilla in a large attractively-shaped glass. Think of it as your Micro Diet cocktail, and serve chilled, or mixed with crushed ice. Sip your Micro Diet through a straw!

Formula for success

There are many, many ways of mixing the eight basic Micro Diet drinks and soups using a great variety of other ingredients. You can experiment yourself, producing different meals to suit your own palate using, for instance, low-calorie soft drinks or flavourings. If you don't mind a few extra calories you can use orange juice, skimmed milk, cocoa, yoghurt or fruit. In fact, anything you want. Have fun and be inventive. To get you started there are suggestions from Uni-Vite's staff dietitians at the end of this chapter.

There are many calorie permutations using The Micro Diet and The Micro Meal to enable you to ring the changes from day to day – for there is much more to the Uni-Vite slimming plans than the *rapid* loss programme of 330 calories a day. But let's begin with the ultimate slimming method that has excited so many Micro-Dieters.

The 330 plan`

The Micro Diet formula   3 servings = 110 calories each

Example
Breakfast: Hot Chocolate
Lunch: Strawberry
Dinner: Chicken & Herb soup

The simple mathematical equation is that 3,500 calories equals 1 lb. of fat. Many women would normally consume at least 1,800–2,000 calories a day so $2,000 - 330 = 1,670$ calories saved (or ½ lb. in weight lost). Hence, this rapid weight loss plan should result in a weight loss of 1 lb. every two days.

All of your essential daily nutritional requirements are concentrated into three Micro Diet servings. In addition it is essential to drink plenty of fluids while on the diet – at least three to four pints, preferably of water. Unsweetened black coffee and lemon tea are alternatives while diet soft drinks (one cal.) can also be consumed but should be used with caution because their sodium content can lead to water retention.

Clinical trials have proved that people with a real need to lose weight (at least two stone) can use a Very Low Calorie Diet for extended periods of time. **We strongly recommend, however, that The Micro Diet be used as your sole source of nutrition for no more than three weeks at a**

time. During the fourth week, one low-calorie meal of solid food a day is added to the three Micro Diet meals as part of our programme to improve your regular eating habits.

As long as you still have fat stores to burn up, this 'three weeks-one week' pattern can be observed until you reach your target weight. The 'sole source' regime is not designed for those people who simply want to lose a few pounds to improve their appearance.

The 420 and 440 plans

Men, whose energy and protein requirements are generally greater than those of women, should follow one of these plans as their minimum intake. These regimes are also more suitable for anyone performing heavy physical tasks or exercising regularly. It would also make sense for someone who might be hungry during the first few days to enjoy an extra serving of The Micro Diet rather than snacking on anything else. Quite often, Micro-Dieters find that they prefer to have half portions of the formula (with the full amount of liquid) and therefore enjoy six or eight 'meals' spaced throughout the course of the day.

(420) The Micro Diet formula	3 servings: 2 mixed with water = 110 calories each, 1 mixed with skimmed milk = 200 calories

Example

Breakfast:	Banana/water
Lunch:	Beef soup
Dinner:	Vanilla/skimmed milk

(440) The Micro Diet formula	4 servings: all with water = 110 calories each

Example

Breakfast:	Chocolate
Lunch:	Strawberry
Early evening:	Chicken and Herb soup
Late evening:	Butterscotch

The 470 plan

This plan is perfectly suited for anyone 'on the move'. It involves substituting a Micro Meal bar for one of the formula meals. The bar contains only 140 calories more than the normal drink plan but has the double bonus of extra protein and a substantial supply of fibre. It also satisfies the need for 'something to chew'.

The Micro Diet formula   2 servings = 110 calories each
The Micro Meal bar   1 serving = 250 calories

Example
Breakfast: Coffee
Lunch: Micro Meal bar
Dinner: Hot Chocolate

The 510 plan

The Micro Diet formula   3 servings: 2 with approx. ½ oz. of skimmed milk powder added = 400 calories, 1 with water only = 110 calories

Example
Breakfast: Chocolate with skimmed milk
Lunch: Chicken & Herb soup
Dinner: Strawberry with skimmed milk

Obviously you can vary the theme depending on individual lifestyle, personal preferences and nutritional demands. Here are some more possibilities to build slightly higher caloric intakes.

The 560 plan

| The Micro Diet formula | 2 servings: 1 with skimmed milk = 200 calories, 1 with water = 110 calories |
| The Micro Meal bar | 1 serving = 250 calories |

Example

Breakfast:	Banana
Lunch:	Micro Meal bar
Dinner:	Vanilla with skimmed milk

The 600 plan

| The Micro Diet formula | 3 servings: all mixed with skimmed milk = 200 calories each |

The 610 plan

| The Micro Diet formula | 1 serving = 110 calories |
| The Micro Meal bar | 2 servings = 250 calories each |

The 650 plan

| The Micro Diet formula | 2 servings with skimmed milk = 200 calories each |
| The Micro Meal bar | 1 serving = 250 calories |

The 700 plan

| The Micro Diet formula | 1 serving with skimmed milk = 200 calories |
| The Micro Meal bar | 2 servings = 250 calories each |

The 750 plan

| The Micro Meal bar | 3 servings = 250 calories each |

Total Nutritional Profile

PLANS	Protein (g)	Carbohydrates (g)	Fat (g)	Vitamins	Minerals	Trace Elements	Electrolytes
330	42	35.1	3.0	100%	100%	100%	100%
*420	51.3	48.7	3.27	At least 100%	At least 100%	At least 100%	At least 100%
440	56	46.8	4.0	At least 100%	At least 100%	At least 100%	At least 100%
470	43	61.6	7.1	100%	100%	100%	100%
510	60.5	62.4	3.5	At least 100%	At least 100%	At least 100%	At least 100%
560	52.3	75.2	7.4	At least 100%	At least 100%	At least 100%	At least 100%
600	69.8	76	3.8	At least 100%	At least 100%	At least 100%	At least 100%
610	44	88.1	11.2	100%	100%	100%	100%
650	61.5	88.9	7.6	At least 100%	At least 100%	At least 100%	At least 100%
700	53.3	101.7	11.5	At least 100%	At least 100%	At least 100%	At least 100%
750	45	114.6	15.3	100%	100%	100%	100%

Percentage of recommended Daily Allowance recognised by either: W.H.O., D.H.S.S., American Academy of Science, D.G.E. (German Nutritional Society).

* Recommended starting point for men.

Alternatively, of course, the slimmer can benefit from replacing two ordinary meals a day with the excellent nutritional base of two Micro Diet meals and having a sensible ordinary meal at whichever time of day suits them. We recommend some low-calorie (approx. 400 calorie) meals in Part II of this book.

All of the plans are designed to give you all the nutrition you need. Page 43 shows what each plan contains.

Dear Sir/Madam,

The Micro Diet has made me a 'normal' human being again. Before the Diet I was becoming a neurotic and very morose person. I used to snap at anyone who mentioned the word weight. I wouldn't go out to places where I thought people who didn't know me would see me. I spent last summer mainly in jumpers to hide myself, especially on the beach. I had to go out sometimes because my children (now aged 4 yrs and 2 yrs) wanted to swim. If I could, I got out of it by sending my husband. I wouldn't buy clothes because I was ashamed of my size. Any new clothes I had were made for me and I looked continually pregnant. I used to be a size 18 – mainly 20. Now I can wear some of my old size 14 clothes, but I'm mainly a size 16. I've even bought a pair of trousers! The first pair in 8 years.

I've had medical help, medication, strict medical diets, but no matter how long the course of tablets or diets lasted, I never lost more than 10 lbs. With the Micro Diet, in 3 months I went from 15 st. 7 lb. to 12 st. 3 lb., and now I'm trying to lose the last 16 lb. to reach my ideal weight for my height, which is 11 st. 7 lb. My husband says he's got back the girl he asked to marry him, my family say I'm the old Karen again, and my dad, he just says, 'Hello Slim Jim.' Even my son says 'Mummy looks nice.'

This summer it's a new swimsuit for me and down to the beach, and I don't care who sees me.

Thank you Micro Diet. I can get back to living

again instead of hiding. Playing with my children outside instead of only indoors. My family are all proud of me and my achievement, but most important of all, I'm proud of myself.

I no longer cry myself to sleep, or mind seeing my reflection in a mirror. In fact I've been doing a lot of that lately. Seeing how I look in my new clothes.

If *I* can do it, anyone can.

Yours sincerely,

Karen Murray
Bognor Regis
W. Sussex.

The food diary

Keeping a daily record of what you eat and drink will help you to become more aware of your personal eating habits.

Use this chart even if you are embarking on the 'sole source' nutrition plan as it will be visible testimony to your progress. Continue filling in the diary while following the maintenance programme or the lifetime nutrition plan.

Tick the boxes each time you have a Micro Diet drink or Micro Meal and, in the space provided, write 'other' food and drink which you may consume. Ideally, note down the time and 'reason'. Did you have that chocolate biscuit at 3 p.m. because you were really hungry? Or because you were just bored, angry, upset or anxious . . .?

Enter a cross at the times you are hungry so that after a week you can adjust meal times accordingly.

Very often we are unaware of why we overeat. Keeping a daily record will reveal your personal eating pattern. Once you have identified that pattern and the reason behind it you are already on the road to healthier eating. Alternatively, you may be surprised to discover that even though you don't consume very much, those extra inches refuse to disappear. It could be that you have a low metabolic rate, making it all the more important to be faithful to the 330-a-day plan.

Write down everything that you eat . . . that lump of cheese, that handful of peanuts. You may be astonished at the amount of calories consumed while driving the car, watching television, or even chatting on the telephone. Don't cheat by not writing it all down because in the end you are only cheating yourself.

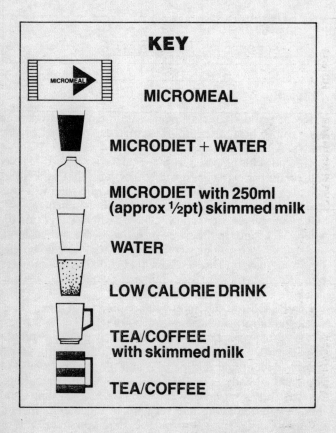

KEY

MICROMEAL

MICRODIET + WATER

MICRODIET with 250ml (approx ½pt) skimmed milk

WATER

LOW CALORIE DRINK

TEA/COFFEE with skimmed milk

TEA/COFFEE

DAILY FOOD DIARY

	MONDAY	TUESDAY	NOTES
7am–11am BREAKFAST	▼ ☐ MICRODIET MICRODIET ▶ ☐	▼ ☐ MICRODIET MICRODIET ▶ ☐	
11am–3pm LUNCH	▼ ☐ MICRODIET MICRODIET ▶ ☐	▼ ☐ MICRODIET MICRODIET ▶ ☐	
3pm–7pm EVENING MEAL	▼ ☐ MICRODIET MICRODIET ▶ ☐	▼ ☐ MICRODIET MICRODIET ▶ ☐	
7pm–12pm			
MICRODIET plus daily liquid intake	☐☐☐☐☐ ☐☐☐☐☐ ☐☐☐☐☐ ☐☐☐☐☐ ☐☐☐☐☐ ☐☐☐☐☐	☐☐☐☐☐ ☐☐☐☐☐ ☐☐☐☐☐ ☐☐☐☐☐ ☐☐☐☐☐ ☐☐☐☐☐	

DAILY FOOD DIARY

	WEDNESDAY	THURSDAY	FRIDAY
7am–11am BREAKFAST	MICRODIET	MICRODIET	MICRODIET
11am–3pm LUNCH	MICRODIET	MICRODIET	MICRODIET
3pm–7pm EVENING MEAL	MICRODIET	MICRODIET	MICRODIET
7pm–12pm			
MICRODIET plus daily liquid intake			

DAILY FOOD DIARY

	SATURDAY	SUNDAY	NOTES
7am–11am BREAKFAST	■ □ MICRODIET ▶ □	■ □ MICRODIET ▶ □	
11am–3pm LUNCH	■ □ MICRODIET ▶ □	■ □ MICRODIET ▶ □	
3pm–7pm EVENING MEAL	■ □ MICRODIET ▶ □	■ □ MICRODIET ▶ □	
7pm–12pm			
MICRODIET plus daily liquid intake	■ □	■ □	

Ringing the changes

No matter how much you might like the chocolate, you won't want to drink it 'neat' three times a day, seven days a week! Here are some appetising ideas from Uni-Vite's dietitians.

Butterscotch

Brandy Butter
One serving Butterscotch Uni-Vite
½ tsp. brandy essence
250ml. (½ pint) cold water

Old English Butterscotch
One serving Butterscotch Uni-Vite
¼–½ tsp. nutmeg
250ml. (½ pint) cold water

Tropical Butterscotch
One serving Butterscotch Uni-Vite
¼ Ogen melon puréed
250ml. (½ pint) cold water

Butternut
One serving Butterscotch Uni-Vite
¼ tsp. coconut essence
250ml. (½ pint) cold water

Vanilla

Cola Shake
One serving Vanilla Uni-Vite
½ pint Diet Coke

Frozen Daiquiri
One serving Vanilla Uni-Vite
½ tsp. rum essence
Crushed ice and Diet Lemon and Lime

Orange Fizz
One serving Vanilla Uni-Vite
Orangeade
Water to taste

Shandy Shake
One serving Vanilla Uni-Vite
Shandy/water mixed

Tangerine Dream
One serving Vanilla Uni-Vite
¼ tsp. tangerine flavouring
250ml. (½ pint) cold water

Apricot Delight
One serving Vanilla Uni-Vite
¼ tsp. Apricot flavouring
Cinnamon
250ml. (½ pint) cold water

Pineapple Cream
One serving Vanilla Uni-Vite
¼ tsp. pineapple flavouring
250ml. (½ pint) cold water

Eastern Promise
One serving Vanilla Uni-Vite
¼ tsp. rose essence
250ml. (½ pint) cold water

Caribbean Cocktail
One serving Vanilla Uni-Vite
4 drops coconut essence
4 drops pineapple essence
250ml. (½ pint) cold water

Beef

Beef and Tomato Soup
One serving Beef Uni-Vite
1 tsp. tomato purée
250ml. (½ pint) hot water

Beef and Herb Soup
One serving Beef Uni-Vite
½ tsp. mixed herb purée
250ml. (½ pint) hot water

Chilli Beef
One serving Beef Uni-Vite
4 drops tabasco
250ml. (½ pint) hot water

Savoury Beef Soup
One serving Beef Uni-Vite
¼ oxo cube
250ml. (½ pint) hot water

Provençale Soup
One serving Beef Uni-Vite
½ tsp. garlic purée
250ml. (½ pint) hot water

Devilled Beef
One serving Beef Uni-Vite
½ tsp. tomato purée
¼ tsp. cayenne pepper
250ml. (½ pint) hot water

Peppered Beef
One serving Beef Uni-Vite
Ground black pepper to taste
250ml. (½ pint) hot water

Chicken and Herb

Thick Curried Chicken
One serving Chicken and
Herb Uni-Vite
¼ tsp. curry powder
½ tsp. turmeric
2 drops liquid sweetener
250ml. (½ pint) hot water

Chicken Worcester
One serving Chicken and
Herb Uni-Vite
½ tsp. Worcester Sauce
½ tsp. onion powder
250ml. (½ pint) hot water

Chinese Chicken Soup
One serving Chicken and
Herb Uni-Vite
½ tsp. Soy sauce
Chopped beansprouts
250ml.(½ pint) hot water

Hungarian Chicken
One serving Chicken and
Herb Uni-Vite
½ tsp. paprika
½ tsp. garlic purée
250ml. (½ pint) hot water

Spring Chicken
One serving Chicken and
Herb Uni-Vite
½ tsp. dried chives
1 stalk chopped parsley
250ml.(½ pint) hot water

Middle East Chicken
One serving Chicken and
Herb Uni-Vite
½ tsp. coriander
½ tsp. garlic purée
250ml. (½ pint) hot water

Chicken and Vegetable Soup
One serving Chicken and
Herb Uni-Vite
½ stick celery
1 small grated carrot
¼ tsp. onion powder
250ml. (½ pint) hot water

Peking Chicken
One serving Chicken and
Herb Uni-Vite
¼ tsp. ginger
½ tsp. garlic purée
½ tsp. chives
250ml. (½ pint) hot water

Coffee

Coffee Marzipan
One serving Coffee Uni-Vite
¼ tsp. almond essence
250ml. (½ pint) hot water

Neopolitan Coffee
One serving Coffee Uni-Vite
½ tsp. vanilla essence
250ml. (½ pint) chilled water

Cool Tipsy Coffee
One serving Coffee Uni-Vite
½ tsp. rum essence
½ tsp. brandy essence
250ml. (½ pint) chilled water

Hot Mocha
One serving Coffee Uni-Vite
1½ tsp. drinking chocolate
250ml. (½ pint) hot water

Strong Iced Coffee
One serving Coffee Uni-Vite
1 tsp. coffee powder
250ml. (½ pint) chilled water

Strawberry

Butterberry
½ serving Butterscotch
Uni-Vite
½ serving Strawberry Uni-Vite
250ml. (½ pint) cold water

Caribbean Strawberry
One serving Strawberry
Uni-Vite
¼ tsp. rum essence
250ml. (½ pint) cold water

Sunny Strawberry Delight
One serving Strawberry
Uni-Vite
1 tbs. raspberries
250ml. (½ pint) cold water

Strawberry Zest
One serving Strawberry
Uni-Vite
Grated zest of ½ lemon
250ml. (½ pint) cold water

Strawberry Fizz
One serving Strawberry
Uni-Vite
½ pint Diet 7-Up

South Sea Strawberry
One serving Strawberry
Uni-Vite
½ juice from lime
250ml. (½ pint) cold water

Banana

Chocolate Banana
½ serving Banana Uni-Vite
½ serving Chocolate Uni-Vite
250ml. (½ pint) cold water

Cinnamon Banana
One serving Banana Uni-Vite
¼ tsp. ground cinnamon
250ml. (½ pint) cold water

Spicy Banana
One serving Banana Uni-Vite
¼ tsp. mixed spice
250ml. (½ pint) hot water

Banana Split
One serving Banana Uni-Vite
1½ tsp. drinking chocolate
250ml. (½ pint) cold water

Banana Supreme
One serving Banana Uni-Vite
½ puréed banana
250ml. (½ pint) cold water

Gingered Banana
One serving Banana Uni-Vite
⅓–½ tsp. banana essence
250ml. (½ pint) cold water

Old English Banana
One serving Banana Uni-Vite
⅓ – ½ tsp. nutmeg
250ml. (½ pint) cold water

Jamaica Banana
One serving Banana Uni-Vite
½ tsp. coconut essence
250ml. (½ pint) cold water

Chocolate

Hot Milk Chocolate
½ serving Chocolate Uni-Vite
½ serving Vanilla Uni-Vite
250ml. (½ pint) hot water

Chocolate Cola
One serving Chocolate
Uni-Vite
½ pint Diet Coke or Diet Cola
Water to taste

Cool Chocolate Mint
One serving Chocolate
Uni-Vite
¼ tsp. peppermint essence
250ml. (½ pint) cold water

Chocolate Orange Supreme
One serving Chocolate
Uni-Vite
¼ tsp. orange
250ml. (½ pint) cold water

Coconana
One serving Chocolate
Uni-Vite
¼ tsp. coconut essence
250ml. (½ pint) cold water

5

THE EVIDENCE

Half a million people can't be wrong! The practical experience throughout Britain speaks volumes for The Micro Diet – both the product and the programme.

The Uni-Vite survey

Word of mouth reports about the success of The Micro Diet were tremendously exciting. We heard, for example, about rapid weight losses, specific health improvements or how valuable the support of the Uni-Vite Advisor had been. But it was not until Dr Jacqueline Stordy at Surrey University's Department of Biochemistry undertook a nationwide survey that we discovered just how unbelievably successful The Micro Diet had been.

In spring of 1985 Dr Stordy randomly distributed an extensive questionnaire to a number of Uni-Vite Advisors. The Advisors, in turn, handed the questionnaire to every third client commencing their third (or more) week on the diet. The clients then returned the completed questionnaires to Dr Stordy.

There were 855 respondents (88.5% women, average age 41), producing some highly illuminating results.

A total of 67% said that they had discovered The Micro Diet through the word of mouth recommendation of a relative, friend or acquaintance while 5.4% had been encouraged to use the diet by a health professional. Not surprisingly, as many slimmers pursue 14 diets during the course of a lifetime, 95% of those surveyed said that they had tried other methods of losing weight. The majority had simply cut calories and 38% had invested money in commercial slimming establishments.

A STAGGERING 94% FOUND IT EASIER TO LOSE WEIGHT WITH UNI-VITE THAN OTHER METHODS.

Quite importantly, the slimmer's family turned out to be more supportive of their weight loss efforts with The Micro Diet than with other methods . . . 75% as opposed to 53%, actually provided 'active encouragement'. The reason for this was not elicited in the survey but it certainly will confound the critics who believe an 'unnatural' liquid-only plan to be socially disruptive. We can only presume that the slimmer was enjoying success, becoming happier, and as a result the family rallied round in support!

Other support and encouragement, of course, is given by the Uni-Vite Advisor and we were delighted to note that 77% of the survey group felt that the role of the Advisor had been either 'very important' or 'fairly important' in helping them achieve their weight loss.

Most of the respondents were still on the weight loss path and incredibly motivated, since 96.4% said that they believed they would reach their target through The Micro Diet. Those slimmers who had achieved their goal were asked the all important question about keeping the weight off.

86% FOUND IT 'EASY' OR 'EASIER' TO MAINTAIN THEIR TARGET WEIGHT WITH UNI-VITE.

A total of 89% of the respondents were continuing to use The Micro Diet as an implicit part of their weight maintenance programme while 76.7% said that their dietary habits had changed since taking The Micro Diet formula.

This statistic is particularly significant as one of the primary criticisms of Very Low Calorie Diets is that they don't teach long-term eating habits. The reality is obviously quite the reverse. There is much more to The

Micro Diet than a powdered formula aiding rapid weight loss but some of the critics are either ignorant of, or choose to ignore, the fact that The Micro Diet is also a lifetime plan for weight maintenance. More often than not, a successful slimmer, after a complete break from ordinary food, becomes acutely aware of the 'bad' foods and is anxious to maintain the new physique gained through The Uni-Vite programme.

Not everyone, of course, embarks on The Micro Diet 'sole source' . . . just 40.5% of those in the survey. Of these people 33% said that they had sought their doctor's approval. Quite frankly, this is a figure which we feel has been improved in the last few months and we would like to see it higher still as . . .

71% OF THOSE DOCTORS ASKED 'ACTIVELY EN-COURAGED' WEIGHT LOSS WITH THE MICRO DIET.

We strongly urge *anyone* wishing to start The Micro Diet to check with their doctor first so that he or she can monitor your progress and form a first-hand appreciation of the benefits of the Uni-Vite plans.

During the course of the diet regime most slimmers – 97.2% had no need at all to consult their doctor with any symptoms. A small number of dieters experienced minor temporary problems (most easily remedied by drinking more water) such as headaches, constipation, dizziness, bad breath and hunger. The vast majority, however, commented on improvements in their sense of well-being.

89% 'FELT WELL' ON THE DIET, 71% NOTICED HEALTH IMPROVEMENT.

Additionally the slimmers were asked about the flavours available to them. A total of 91% said they liked the taste 'very much' or found it to be 'quite nice' or 'acceptable'. At that time there were only five Uni-Vite flavours available: Vanilla, Strawberry, Chocolate, Butterscotch and Chicken & Herb. The range now, of course, includes Banana, Coffee and Beef soup.

Says Dr Stordy, Senior Lecturer in Nutrition, 'The results from the survey were very impressive. It is obvious that a great many people have clearly benefited from their experience with The Micro Diet.'

Before the public experience, of course, had to come the clinical trials. There were wide ranging studies with a variety of very low-calorie formulation conducted at many universities and hospitals over the last few years – many are summarised at the end of this chapter. Though the results have been overwhelmingly positive, we decided that specific trials with Uni-Vite's Micro Diet formulation would contribute to the present state of knowledge. Subsequently, studies have been performed at the University of Surrey and the University of Utrecht. The Surrey study showed average weight losses of 16 lb. a month and led Dr Stordy to observe, 'Patients enjoy a sense of well-being . . . their weight loss is so rewarding. It doesn't take a lifetime to lose a substantial amount. A Very Low Calorie Diet is not restrictive. The patients don't generally feel hungry. The Micro Diet actually gives them a sense of freedom because you can go out and enjoy yourself socially or for business . . . and then go back on the diet and quickly start losing again. This diet is the answer for anyone who has had real difficulty losing weight . . .'

Dr Stordy's comments are echoed by the medical doctor who supervised the trial.

Dr John Wright, Reader in Metabolic Medicine at the University: 'I have no hesitation in saying that for people with a low metabolic rate this is an extremely effective and, above all, realistic new approach.'

The trial at the University of Utrecht was deliberately only conducted on slightly overweight women and still showed an average weight loss of 11 lb. in 14 days.

Says Dr Anton Beynen, who carried out the study, 'A well formulated Very Low Calorie Diet regime such as The Micro Diet is undoubtedly the diet of the future. It solves all the previous problems because patients lose weight fast enough to be encouraged and they feel very well at the same time. The time to teach people how to eat

better and cook sensibly is after they have lost weight –
any other approach is normally unrealistic.'

A further clinical trial has been conducted in West
Germany on a Uni-Vite – Micro Diet formula of 600
calories per day. Yet the weight loss was still an impressive 19 lb. over the 28-day trial period, says Dr Alfred
Wirth, head of State Clinic, Teutoburger Wald, former
head of the Heart Research Unit, University of
Heidelberg. From the safety point of view, another recent
German study produced some stunning evidence to show
that *weight is lost on VLCDs in the same way as it is
gained*! Major researcher Professor Ditschuneit of Ulm
University, West Germany, has proven that when weight
is lost on a VLCD the loss was 79% fat, 18% water and
3% protein. This is significant because when weight is
gained, an average 75% of the gain is fat, 19% is water
and 6% extra protein. Some protein loss is inevitable
since, for example, the slimmer's skin is smaller but this
loss is in the expected amount.

A recent VLCD study at the Dept. of Endocrinology,
Metabolism and Nutrition, at the University of Antwerp,
is of particular interest to men on The Micro Diet, since it
was conducted on the same balance of protein and
nutrients as we recommend for men. The study surveyed a
500-calorie formula diet using 60g protein per day, and it
showed 31.7 lb. weight loss over 6 weeks – *21 lb. per 4
weeks*! 'A highly significant decrease could be observed
for body weight, body mass index (−5.2) and fat weight,
*whereas lean body mass and arm muscle circumference
remained unchanged*.'

The objective of any diet must be to produce fast,
encouraging weight loss, but this must be fat loss not
muscle loss.

VLCDs have been shown to achieve this objective.

Talking to your doctor

We are all unique individuals. We cannot personally
monitor you, and you should not assume that because

there is so much evidence to support The Micro Diet that it is automatically perfect for you. It is a fundamental to the Uni-Vite Programme that you involve your doctor. He can advise you whether you should lose weight at the fastest rate (on 330 calories a day during the initial phase) or should add some calories to your three servings of The Micro Diet.

It will help him considerably if you fill in the following questionnaire before your visit. At the same time show your doctor the letter which appears in Appendix B at the end of this book. The questionnaire will inform your doctor as to some of the physical and psychological causes of your overweight, and that in turn will enable him to use the Uni-Vite programme to your best personal advantage.

ANSWER THESE QUESTIONS
BEFORE YOU VISIT YOUR DOCTOR

1. What age were you when you initially became overweight? ....
2. Why do you think you became over-weight? ....
3. How much did you weigh at 21? ....
4. What is the maximum weight you have been? ....
5. Are any of your family overweight? Who? ....
6. Is there any history of diabetes, heart disease or blood pressure in your family? ....
7. Why do you want to lose weight?
    (a) Are you upset at your appearance? ....
    (b) Do you get breathless? ....
    (c) Do you ever feel dizzy? ....
8. What is the weight you want to be? ....
9. Have you tried to lose weight before? ....
10. Would you describe yourself as happy? ....
    (a) Do you ever get tense? ....
    (b) Do you have any particular worries currently? ....
11. How many meals do you eat per day? ....
    (a) Do you eat between meals? ....
    (b) Do you prefer savoury or sweet foods? ....
    (c) Do you take sugar in tea/coffee? ....
    (d) How much alcohol do you drink per day on average? ....
    (e) Do you always eat sitting down? ....
    (f) Do you sometimes eat and do other things e.g. watch TV, read? ....
    (g) Do you eat when you are worried or bored? ....
12. What sort of work do you do? ....
13. How many minutes do you walk a day? ....

60

14. Do you have any active hobbies or play any sport?   ....

15. How many cigarettes do you smoke daily?   ....

16. What is your current weight?   ....

Very low calorie diets

A summary of the main studies

Main Researcher	Sample Size	Diet Studied	Results
1. Prof. Ditschuneit, Ulm University	5,000	VLCDs ranging from 30g to 50g per day of protein in calorie levels from 300–500 kcal.	Av. weight loss of 18 lb. per month. Weight was lost in the proportions: 79% fat, 18% water, 3% protein. This is significant because when weight is gained, on average 75% is fat, 19% is water, and 6% is extra protein. So protein loss is inevitable (e.g. the slimmer's skin is smaller) but is in the expected proportion. *Conclusion* Safe and highly effective.
2. Prof. Apfelbaum, Univ. of Paris	5,000	VLCDs ranging from 300–400 calories Protein 55g to 70g.	No mortality or serious effects despite the fact that the *expected* death rate amongst 5,000 obese people as calculated by Vertes would normally be approx. 0.4% or 20 people, i.e. the VLCD *decreased* the incidence of expected problems.

3.	Vertes, Genuth, Hazelton, Univ. of Cleveland	519	300 Calories 45g Protein 30g Carbohydrate	Av. monthly loss of 13.2 lb. over an entire continuous 29-week period. 78% of patients lost at least 40 lb. *Conclusion* 'An effective means of achieving substantial weight loss rapidly and safely'.
4.	Hickey, Daly et al., St Vincent's Hospital, Dublin	23	320 Calories 30g Protein 45g Carbohydrate	Av. weight loss 17.4 lb. a month. 60% adherence, no serious side effects.
5.	Mancini, Di Biase, Contaldo, Univ. of Naples	389	Various levels including 80, 180, 330, and 360 calories.	Up to 22 lb. per month in initial phase. General beneficial reduction in blood pressure, triglyceride levels and cholesterol levels. After 12–15 months average weight reduction was still 40 lb.
6.	Palgi, Greenberg et al., unpublished	668	450 Calories 80g Protein 10g Carbohydrate	Av. weight loss 46 lb. (11 lb. per month). No serious arrythmia, no mortality.
7.	Phinney, Bistrain, Blackburn et al., New England Hospital, Boston & M.I.T.	13	Two 450 calorie diets. 24 hr. 'holter' E.C.G. monitor to specifically check safety against Liquid Protein Diets.	Weight loss of 17 lb. per 4 weeks. *No* change in ectopic beat frequency. No change in cardiac rhythms.

8.	Genuth, Vertes et al., Mount Sinai Hospital, Cleveland	75	300 Calories 45g Protein 30g Carbohydrate	Av. weight loss of 15.4 lb. per month, over 21-week average diet period. No significant adverse effects. However, beneficial effect in reduction of blood pressure and serum cholesterol noted.
9.	McLean, Baird, West Middlesex Hospital, London	44	320 Calories 31g Protein 44g Carbohydrate	Nitrogen balance reached in 5–6 weeks. No E.C.G. abnormalities. *Conclusion* 'Safe and effective method of outpatient weight reduction'.
10.	Beynen & Gundlach, Utrecht	5	330 Calories 42g Protein 35g Carbohydrate 14 days study on *non-obese* women	Av. weight loss 11.4 lb. in 14 days. 75% of weight loss was adipose tissue. *Conclusion* 'Lean body mass is for the most part spared'.
11.	Rahman, Wright & Stordy	9	330 Calories 42g Protein 35g Carbohydrate 4 Weeks	16 lb. per month weight loss. No E.C.G. abnormalities. No side effects.
12.	Van Gaal, Snyders, de Leevw	15	500 Calories 60g Protein 54g Carbohydrate 6-week study	Weight loss 21 lb. per 4 weeks. Weight loss came almost entirely from consumption of body fat: lean body mass remained unchanged.

| 13. | Amatruda,
Biddle,
Patton,
Lockwood | 6 | 472 Calories
69g Protein
31g Carbo-
hydrate

Test to
measure safety
of nutritionally
complete diets
v. the Liquid
Protein Diet. | 17 lb. per month weight loss. Nitrogen balance achieved after 21 days. No cardiac arrhythmia. |
| 14. | Hoffer,
Bistrian,
Young &
Blackburn | 8 | Two 500
calorie diets

(a) 85g
Protein
0g
Carbo-
hydrate
23g Fat

(b) 44g
Protein
38g
Carbo-
hydrate
18g Fat

Test to see
which diet
produced
nitrogen
equilibrium.
8-week study. | Av. weight loss: 18.0 lb. per month. The high-protein diet produced nitrogen equilibrium; the mixed diet produced a 2g per day nitrogen loss. |

6

THE UNI-VITE ADVISOR

The exceptional nutritional content of The Micro Diet in a mere 330 calories is the tool to help you fashion a new body. But you need a skilled worker to help you use that tool to the best possible effect. That's where the human element is all important – the support and encouragement of an Independent Uni-Vite Advisor.

Certainly, you can follow the diet plans 'in splendid isolation' and *succeed*. But studies have shown that a slimmer's chances of success are greatly improved if they have the benefit of a support system. There is now an army of 15,000 Uni-Vite Advisors throughout the country who can counsel you in the best possible way – through their own personal experience. They have all become Advisors after realising the benefits of the programme themselves. They are able to say 'I've tried it . . . and it works,' and they are able to answer your basic questions. Some of them are trained health professionals; most are not. They are not, of course, expected to replace the role of a doctor or dietitian but to be a 'helping hand' working in conjunction with the qualified practitioner.

The Advisor has the time to spend with the overweight person in whatever way the slimmer chooses – yet another example of the flexibility of the Uni-Vite programme.

Too good to be true

In many parts of the country there are complimentary group meetings where talks are given about the ways of using The Micro Diet and dieters are able to share their experiences. The mutual support and spirit of togetherness generated at such meetings can often be the decisive factor influencing a slimmer to make the first step of actually starting the diet.

We remember vividly one typical Micro Diet meeting held in a small church meeting room in a suburb of Birmingham. It was the middle of winter and only about 20 people had turned out. There were a handful of Advisors, some people in the middle of the diet plan and others who were hearing about the programme for the first time. We discussed how Very Low Calorie Diets had been devised and developed. We talked about the fact that some people just cannot lose weight on 1,000 calories a day and explained that the VLCD offered real hope for such people. We related some of the success stories we had already heard. There was one very large lady listening most attentively, frequently nodding her head in agreement with the points we were making. She seemed to have no doubts about the logic of the VLCD. She had come to the meeting, however, with a skinny friend, presumably for moral support. At the end of the presentation, after we had thanked everyone for attending, the skinny friend exclaimed loudly, 'Bah! Sounds too good to be true!'

Before we had a chance to respond, a woman sitting behind tapped the skinny one on the shoulder and said, to our delight, 'That's exactly what I said two months and two stone ago.' The cloud of doubt which had passed over the face of the large lady disappeared instantly.

It was not the first nor the last time we heard such scepticism. We understand the scepticism. After all, we were once sceptics ourselves. Moreover, the person about to embark on a weight loss regime is setting off on a meaningful journey. The final destination is their ideal body weight and nothing can be more important than their own health and well-being.

They have every right to be sceptical. The likelihood is extremely high that they have already tried many different ways of losing weight. They have already experienced the misery of slow dispiriting weight loss, of giving up in failure or, if they were among the few to reach goal weight, found that the fat came piling back on. To be told that weight losses of 16–20 lb. a month can be achieved while obtaining complete nutrition in a mere 330 calories – and without feeling hungry – certainly does sound too good to be true. Attendance at meetings such as the one in Birmingham is purely on a voluntary basis.

Perhaps instead you would prefer the Advisor to visit you in your home for a small group meeting or a personal chat?

Or perhaps you would like to keep in contact by telephone?

Uni-Vite Advisors are well used to fielding phone calls at home. If it helps to keep you on a continuing weight loss pattern they feel it is time well spent. The Advisor will be happy to help you whichever way you see fit. The praise we have received for the overall quality of the Advisor service is most encouraging.

We've heard about an extremely overweight man in the west of England who was agoraphobic and would not venture outside his front door. Until the Uni-Vite Advisor visited him in the privacy of his own home, he had not felt able to turn to anyone for help. Disabled people have been aided in the same way.

The personal contact is an integral part of the Uni-Vite programme. You, the slimmer, have the example of the Uni-Vite Advisor as a visible sign that the diet plan works. Quite often the Advisor may still be on the weight loss path herself, treading step by step with you.

The Advisor can provide you with the latest Uni-Vite information, whether it is nutritional guidelines, new recipes for mixing the formula, menus of low-calorie solid meals or even new products complementing the existing range. Most of all, though, the Advisor is someone to provide the encouragement and motivation for you to triumph once and for all over your weight problem. We have known all along the immense value to the programme of our Advisors. It was proven in the University of Surrey survey of Uni-Vite slimmers, with 77% describing the role of the Advisors as 'important' or 'fairly important'.

Eminent authorities in the field have also now concluded that such support is an essential part of a successful slimming regime. Dr Denis Craddock, M.D., a member of the Royal College of Physicians Working Party on Obesity, reported in the BMA Slimmer's Guide recently: 'For those who have difficulty in keeping to a diet, groups run by hospitals, family doctors, local authorities and slimming organisations can be valuable'.

World renowned expert Professor A. J. Stunkard of Pennsylvania University, USA, stated in a scientific paper: 'We could make the treatment of obesity more extensive by applying behavioural methods to large populations through the agency of *lay-led* groups'.

Behind the cautious scientific words lies the warmth and emotion of one slimmer helping another towards the same goal.

So often we've heard comments such as, 'I couldn't have made it without my Advisor.'

'I was almost tempted to get stuck into a box of chocolates but I didn't want to let my Advisor down.'

'I was at a really low ebb and then the Uni-Vite meeting gave me all my enthusiasm back.'

The Advisors come from all walks of life: health visitors, nurses and dietitians, for example, who can provide additional insight into the medical and nutritional aspects; but also housewives, secretaries, business executives, engineers and factory workers. All of British society is represented. An Advisor is just a phone call or postcard away. When you are ready, you can obtain the name of your nearest Advisor from this address:

Uni-Vite Nutrition
Station Approach
Great Missenden
Bucks
HP16   OAZ
(02406)   6961

Case history

Name: Susan Corstar
Home town: Abingdon, Oxon.
Weight loss: 2 stone

Doctors refused to set a date for Susan Corstar's major bowel operation because she was too overweight.

Horrified at the prospect of more calorie-counting with little to show for it, Susan, 34, sought solace in more food.

'I was absolutely desperate,' admits Susan, a secretary from Abingdon, Oxon. 'I had tried everything from slimming clubs to "crank" diets and The Micro Diet was my last resort.'

It worked. She lost 2 stone in six weeks reaching her goal of 12 stone, and a date for the operation was set.

Adds Susan: 'Most important to me was the help I received from my Advisor. Whenever I was depressed or tempted to eat, just a phone call away was someone who actually had the same problems and overcame them with Uni-Vite.'

7

WINNERS OUT OF LOSERS

Tons of flab have disappeared since The Micro Diet began making an impact around the country. Office workers in London, farmers in Devon, factory workers in the industrial regions have all forged a common bond: slimming success. And, as a result, they all seem to have become somewhat garrulous . . . they just can't stop talking about the change the diet has made in their lives.

That nationwide success was reflected in the dozens of entries for the first Micro-Dieter of the Year Award, setting the judging panel the arduous task of trying to pick one winner.

In fact, TV and stage actress Diane Keen, star of the series 'Rings on their Fingers', told the audience that many of her showbiz friends were enthusiastic users too, when she made the presentation to the slimming star of 1985, Cornish estate agent John Bray.

There could only be one winner to receive the national award and a cheque for £1,000 but, in his or her own right, everyone losing weight with The Micro Diet is a real winner. Here are some of their stories.

John Bray just cannot believe how he has become a shadow of his former self after losing 6½ stone on The Micro Diet. The 47-year-old estate agent from Rock in Cornwall was so fat he could not swim underwater – he just floated straight to the surface. That was when he weighed in at a hefty 20 st. 4 lb. Now John can swim 60 lengths a day – and stay under as long as he likes.

'Some days I just look at myself in the mirror and cannot believe the man who has emerged from all the blubber,' says John. 'I have got a whole new outlook and whole new lifestyle. It is like being born again.'

John's quest for a new life began with a note of crisis when he collapsed at work with a torn leg muscle brought on by nothing but his excess weight. Doctors warned him that if he didn't lose weight he would spend the rest of his days in a wheelchair.

'I hadn't a clue what to do because I had tried every sort of diet in the world – appetite suppressants, all-fruit diets, salads, special biscuits. You name it and I had tried it. Every one was a disaster. Then someone suggested Uni-Vite's Micro Diet. I just couldn't believe I would make it work as I was always such a big eater. Existing on nothing but three special drinks a day seemed ludicrous,' he candidly recalls. 'It was hard at first, but then I just got to love the stuff.'

John lost a stupendous 30 lb. in the first 21 days and never looked back.

'My doctor, who had supervised it all, is delighted. It has cost me a fortune in buying a new wardrobe but it is worth every penny,' says John.

His wife Annette agrees. 'It's like having a different husband. Not only does he look new and marvellous, he has got energy and zest. And he used to be such a lazy wreck!'

*   *   *

A Manchester couple lost a staggering 16 stone between the two of them!

Ray and Sue Berry, who both work at University Hospital, South Manchester, finally decided to shape up after becoming concerned about their health.

'We both realised that unless we did something to seriously tackle our weight problem, we wouldn't live to see middle age,' says 33-year-old Sue.

It was Ray, though, who embarked on the diet first. When Sue saw the fat melting away at a furious rate she was inspired to follow his example. Ray, a 6'4" X-ray porter, was a colossal 25 stone and shed 10 stone in just 5 months.

'The weight was disappearing so fast that the doctors kept asking me if I was all right,' says Ray. 'Well I am. I have a whole new lease of life.'

Suffering from asthma, Ray's overweight only made things worse. Walking up stairs made him tired and breathless. He remembers, 'I couldn't get on buses easily. I couldn't drive easily. In fact, being so big made everything twice as difficult. Now my lifestyle has changed dramatically. I enjoy going for walks in the country and tending the garden, whereas everyday things had become a chore.'

Says Sue, who got rid of six stone herself, 'It's wonderful to be able to wear my engagement and wedding rings after so long.'

* * *

Among the many letters we receive, this one makes its point so well that we will let Mrs Wasley speak for herself . . .

Dear Uni-Vite,

Last February my husband and I went to Gran Canaria and whilst sitting around the swimming pool the conversation inevitably turned to food and dieting. 'Inevitable' because I was a 13½-stone nurse married to a 17-stone ex-Rugby player, so it was not difficult to see that weight was a problem, especially in swimwear.

One couple showed us a newspaper article describing The Micro Diet which they had started a few weeks previously. To my surprise my husband was very interested and volunteered to join me on The Micro Diet when we returned home.

After six weeks, I am an 11-stone nurse with a 15-stone husband intent on becoming 10- and 14-stone holidaymakers.

Why then did The Micro Diet work where other diets have failed?

There are three reasons. 1. Simplicity: There is no guesswork, calorie counting, weighing food or other complications; just one sachet in eight fluid ounces of water. 2. Flexibility: As a true meal replacement it can adapt to any social pattern. 3. Results: The rapid and consistent weight loss really encourages you to carry on and as your measurements reduce quickly, friends notice and the compliments you receive provide the greatest incentive. So roll on the next holiday when I will truly be able to say: 'I know a diet that really works – The Micro Diet.'

Mrs M. P. Wasley
Puriton,
Bridgwater,
Somerset

*　　*　　*

'I was a shameful size 26 but now I'm proud to say I've shrunk to a trim 16. I no longer need to hide myself under big cardigans and old-fashioned clothes.'

Ten sizes of clothes less also meant more than four stones of weight loss for Jennifer Clements of Aylesbury, Bucks . . . in just three months.

The transformation was so great that when Jennifer returned, after an absence of only a few months, to the Brownie Pack where she had been Brown Owl none of the 24 Brownies or their parents recognised her.

Adds Jennifer, 'I feel like a teenager again.'

*　　*　　*

Bob Wilkins used to wear an overcoat to mow the lawn. Then he took to carrying out the chore under cover of darkness because he couldn't handle the stares of the curious.

For Bob weighed in at a hefty 20 stone and was acutely conscious of the sorry figure he cut. His escape was compulsive eating which, in turn, exacerbated job and personal problems.

Then, 6'3"-tall Bob, of Manchester, discovered The Micro Diet and lost a total of four stone in 3 months.

'I had tried dozens of other diets without success,' he

says, 'but the Uni-Vite diet was different, and the transformation in me has been quite astonishing. During my working day I used to stop off at service stations to buy – and eat – six bars of chocolate. Now I have my eating under control and I'm maintaining my weight. I now feel more confident and can at last enjoy swimming again!'

*　　*　　*

Successful slimmer Joan Day shed 5 stone in just 4½ months to register 9 stone for the first time she can remember.

'I have struggled to lose weight ever since I left school weighing 13½ stone,' confesses the 42-year-old Leeds grandmother. 'But conventional dieting was so slow I always lost heart. With The Micro Diet I shed 1½ stone in the first two weeks. Now I feel great. I haven't felt so fit since I got married 22 years ago.'

Husband Julian is also suitably impressed, saying: 'I feel like I'm married to a new woman.'

*　　*　　*

In the Derby area, Beryl Price got rid of over two stone in five weeks and Margaret Hobbs disposed of three stone in six weeks.

'I'd tried every diet under the sun and been to all the slimming clubs. The Micro Diet was by far the easiest!' says Beryl; while Margaret boasts, 'I can even get into my daughter's trendy clothes – though I'd never wear them in public!'

*　　*　　*

In the Avon area Jean Milton melted away 1½ stone in just seven weeks while husband Roger, not to be outdone, lost two stone in the same period.

'The nutritional value of The Micro Diet was what impressed me most,' says Jean.

*　　*　　*

In Somerset, Vanessa Linnell, of Taunton and her friend Julia Clasby of Bridgwater each got rid of 4 stone.

Tipping the scales at 17 st. 4 lb. after the birth of her second child, Vanessa's midwife recommended The Micro Diet.

'I could hardly believe the results. It took me just 10 weeks to lose the first 3½ stone. But the best thing is the fact that for the first time ever I have been able to maintain my weight loss,' she says.

Julia, who gained a stone with each of her children, took 3 months to lose her weight, and continues to use The Micro Diet for weight maintenance.

'In spite of the very low calorie level I found I had bags of energy. Coping with the children became much easier,' says Julia, who now runs an aerobic class.

∶ *   *   *

Dear Sir,

At last, a diet that works! Over the years I have watched with apathy as my dimensions have steadily increased. At 18 I weighed 6¾ stone and wore size 3½ shoes. Now 20 years later even my foot size has increased to five.

I was spurred into action this Christmas when, in horror, I noticed my weight was 10¾ stone and that my diet of chips and chocolate had taken its toll. Not that my overeating and consequent overweight had gone unnoticed. I have subjected myself of rigorous tortures as an instant answer to dieting.

I have suffered the indignities of being wrapped in bandages, steamy saunas, vitatone massage so vigorous the pain resembled contractions. I even tried eating almost raw pork for a while in order to grow a tape worm to consume some of my extra calories!

I hated being fat. My bra left a huge red weal around my chest and my pants almost stopped the circulation in my legs at the end of the day. My major problem was my faddy food habits: I do not like or eat salads, cheese, fish or much else that is good for me and these foods are always part of a conventional diet. As a fairly keen horsewoman my size was a definite impediment. Apart from the fact that it is not a pretty sight to see pounds of pulsating flesh galloping towards you, the movement of my horse started a chain reaction of spare tyres which bounced from one to another. Who says there is no such thing as perpetual motion?

I was a bit sceptical about The Micro Diet, but – surprise, surprise – it tasted quite palatable, filled me up and for the first time in ages I didn't want a bun for breaktime. Almost at once I noticed that skirts fitted, buttons fastened and blouse buttons stayed done up. I lost 5 lb. in the first week and 6 weeks later I have lost 1 st. 2 lb.

I am not the stuff that Saints and Martyrs are made of, so if I can do it The Micro Diet must be good. It would be a lie to say that a glass of The Micro Diet is as good as a roast meal but it keeps the hunger pangs well at bay. It's easy to mix and shows quick results. All the ingredients added to a small spoonful of will power, and success is yours. I was afraid to tell my friends that I was trying it, as a series of past failures would result in scepticism. Actions speak louder than words and the results have given me confidence to tell people that the new slim me is due entirely to The Micro Diet.

Madelaine Reed
Bridgwater
Somerset

* * *

Slimming with Uni-Vite – The Micro Diet is often a family affair. The Walkers of Whitby, dieted together. David, Eve and son Jonathon, lost seven stone between them in the first three months. Now they share a total weight loss of 11 stone.

Says Eve, who is now more than 4 stone lighter, 'A year ago I was a miserable recluse. I was so self-conscious. I hated going out. I virtually only went out to do the shopping. Now I feel terrific. For months I had existed on cottage cheese and salads without losing weight. In fact, if

I consumed more than 500 calories a day I seemed to gain weight. It took The Micro Diet to do the trick and now I feel terrific.'

*   *   *

The Gardiners, from Abingdon, Oxon, also made a joint slimming effort. Michael, Aline and son Michael all lost two stones each in under seven weeks.

Michael senior, 55, no longer needs to take pain killing drugs for his severe arthritis. 'I'm just amazed and I have so much energy now,' he says.

*   *   *

'Sceptics still scoff, but fans of The Micro Diet just keep losing weight,' said Bournemouth's *Evening Echo* in a story headlined 'A Dieting Revolution'.

Journalists who have tried the diet themselves also end up being convinced.

Martin Howey, for instance, in the *Journal* of Newcastle-upon-Tyne reported: 'Anything that sounded so simple was worth a try. After all, the reluctance of dietitians to come up with anything vaguely uncomplicated was probably the very reason I had never opted to give one a go in the past.

'But here it was. My big chance. The opportunity to lose that half a stone of beer and junk food in a week.

'Prescription: Take three sachets of powder a day and mix with either hot or cold water for all the nutrition the body needs.

'Theory: Excess weight will fall off as will the desire to eat.

'Conclusion: It actually works!

'Seven days later the six pounds which must have cost hundreds of pounds have gone. Just another crash course in dieting? I don't know. It's the only one I have ever been on in my life. But one thing I do know. The Micro Diet works for you. And it doesn't take too much willpower. No one was more sceptical than I.'

Added Martin, 'Having cheated only once, I feel my little box of tricks was money well spent at £10.50 for 21 sachets.'

8

YOUR QUESTIONS ANSWERED

1. *Is it necessary to take additional vitamins while on the Micro Diet plan?*

No! As long as you have at least three servings of the formula you are receiving 100 per cent of the Department of Health's Recommended Daily Amounts. Scientific opinion, in general, decries the use of megadoses of vitamins or other nutrients. However, the choice is yours. If you do wish to supplement your diet, for some specific reason, ask your doctor.

2. *Will everyone lose weight on this diet? I've tried everything and nothing seems to work.*

Yes! Everyone should lose weight with The Micro Diet. The only difference is how much and how fast. No one, over a period of time, can maintain their weight on the rapid weight loss plan of just 330 calories a day. There has to be a continued FAT loss when utilising The Micro Diet as the sole source of nutrition. Nature makes men burn more calories than women; therefore men lose faster.

3. *Why are pregnant women advised not to use the formula?*

Mothers-to-be should plan their diet carefully and always seek their physician's advice. Pregnant women are usually prescribed extra vitamins and it would not be wise to take unnecessary supplements. One daily sachet of The Micro Diet or one Micro Meal food bar can, however, make an extremely valuable contribution to a woman's nutritional needs.

4. *This diet sounds too good to be true. There must be some negative side effects.*

Yes, of course. As with any diet plan your body is undergoing a dramatic change in routine and may react in many different ways. Problems occur for a minority of people, are usually mild and last just a day or two. The long-term benefits make them more than worthwhile.

5. *Headaches for instance?*

Yes. The main reasons could be withdrawal from caffeine to which your body has become addicted, or not taking enough fluid. Drink plenty of water to avoid headaches.

6. *What about dizziness?*

This is most often caused by the diuretic effect that accompanies any low-calorie diet. A reduction in the amount of fluid circulating in the body may result in dizziness, especially when standing up quickly. Solution: drink plenty of fluids and don't stand up quickly.

7. *And nausea?*

Some people will react to the high concentration of nutrients in the formula. This is a very temporary condition. It can be alleviated by drinking six half portions or an extra glass of water with a full sachet. If this is not effective, eat normally, adding the formula as a supplement and then gradually discontinue solid food.

8. *I find that I have bad breath. Why?*

A small number of people complain of halitosis or bad breath. In some cases this may be due to the production of ketones and in others it is caused by a reduction in saliva or the reflux of gas from the stomach. Drinking plenty of fluids speeds up stomach emptying and also helps to wash the mouth.

9. *Will The Micro Diet benefit my arthritis?*

The diet plan will not cure any type of arthritis *but* symptoms in arthritis of the weight-bearing joints will probably be alleviated by the loss of excess weight. Patients frequently report that they are able to decrease the amount of anti-inflammatory drugs. *Some* claim total freedom from any symptoms.

10.   *I have diabetes. Is the diet OK for me?*
Patients with diabetes MUST be under the direct supervision of their physician. A growing number of medical experts, however, familiar with Very Low Calorie Diets, feel that this is the method of choice for the treatment of obese maturity onset diabetes. There are many case histories in which all clinical evidence of diabetes disappears as the patient approaches his ideal weight.

11.   *I don't need to lose weight but I'd like to use the formula meals as a nutritional supplement. What do you recommend?*
In addition to ordinary food, the benefits of taking The Micro Diet, or The Micro Meal, once or twice a day, will make a major contribution to your nutritional needs.

12.   *Why do you recommend drinking so much liquid every day?*
Water is good for you! Our bodies consist of over 60% water, so we need to constantly replace our body fluids. Sufficient liquid intake is also required to keep our kidneys functioning properly, to help prevent constipation and, interestingly, to help prevent fluid retention.

13.   *Could I take the liquid in the form of beer or other kinds of alcohol?*
Only if you want to get drunk really fast! Seriously, alcohol is a major impediment to any diet plan. It contains seven calories per gram compared with four calories per gram of protein or carbohydrate. In fact, it almost holds as many calories as fat, which 'costs' nine calories per gram.

14. *What about coffee?*

Be careful. It's amazing the number of calories you can accumulate if you add milk and sugar. Typically, the addition of milk and two teaspoons of sugar would provide an extra 59 calories.

15. *What about soft drinks?*

Avoid them like the plague! They're full of calories and have little or no nutritional content. A can of coke, for instance, has 130 calories.

16. *Are diet soft drinks permissible then?*

You're on safer ground here. But many contain high amounts of sodium (which causes water retention) and caffeine, so again tread carefully. Be moderate.

17. *Please comment on the level of sodium in the formula itself.*

There are 500 mg of sodium per 100-calorie serving, or 1500 mg per day. This is considered a low sodium regime. Consult your doctor if he has previously placed you on a low sodium diet.

18. *Surely I'll become constipated, only consuming 330 calories a day?*

It depends on what you mean by constipation. As much less bulk is being consumed you should not expect to be as regular as you were before you started the diet programme. This is perfectly normal and no cause for concern. However, it is quite permissible to add bran to your daily intake, always bearing in mind the calories you will also be adding. The problem tends to be worse if sufficient fluid is not consumed so it is important to follow our recommended intake of fluids a day.

19. *Are the nutrients in The Micro Diet synthetic or natural?*

The principal nutrients are obviously natural, coming from milk solids and soybeans. Some of the added vitamins and minerals are 'nature identical', as are many that you find in health food stores. This means that they are manufactured but identical to the chemical composition of the natural element. Your body cannot tell the difference between natural and synthetic nutrients. They are molecularly the same and perform equally well.

20.   *Soon after starting The Micro Diet plan I developed a bad cold. Why was this?*
You caught a cold virus! It's as simple as that. You've had colds in the past and will probably catch a cold in the future. It was just an unfortunate coincidence.

Jill Saville of Lincoln, saved from a painful back operation after losing 3½ stone in 11 weeks, 'I have never felt better in my life . . . nor looked it. My hair, skin and nails are in much better condition. It's marvellous.'

---

21.   *I'm worried that by losing a lot of weight quickly, I will look gaunt and haggard. Are you sure this won't happen?*
On the contrary. Slimmers who lose weight with The Micro Diet not only are healthy, they look healthy – probably because of the fine nutritional content. The drawn look usually occurs when people have been starving themselves or have lost weight through illness. With The Micro Diet you're not depriving yourself of anything – except calories.

22.   *I find it initially hard using The Micro Diet as my 'sole source' of nutrition. Can I take an appetite suppressant to stop my craving solid food?*
It is strongly recommended that you don't. For one thing they can cause unpleasant side effects such as headaches, anxiety and even nausea, and also they are just not necessary. After the first couple of days any mild hunger pangs will disappear.

83

23. *What happens if I can't resist temptation and I 'cheat' while I'm on the diet?*

The Micro Diet is the benevolent diet. Since your basic calorie intake is so low, having a snack or adding a meal will, at worst, halt your weight loss pattern for a day or so. Once you are back on the 'sole source' plan you'll start shedding fat again. Whatever happens, continue with three formula meals every day. As long as you do that, you'll succeed.

24. *Does it matter what time of day I have the three meals?*

It is recommended that you have your three formula meals at regular mealtimes – breakfast, lunch and dinner. This way, your body's nutritional fuel tank is being topped up at measured intervals. Breakfast is particularly important. How many people can say they get one third of their daily nourishment first thing in the morning?

25. *I am taking the birth control pill. Will the diet cause any problems?*

No difficulties have come to light in either the clinical studies or public experience.

26. *My doctor feels that a 330-calorie a day plan is a 'crash' diet and must be a 'fad'. I really want to try it. What can I do?*

Your doctor has a right to be cautious. Your health is in his hands. Most of the research into Very Low Calorie Diets is recent and some of it has yet to find its way into the medical text books. Medical fact sheets have been prepared so that your doctor can familiarise himself with the impressive clinical studies and monitor your progress. You should also show him the letter in Appendix B and the research results in Chapter 5.

27. *Am I more likely to develop infections because of the stress of dieting and consuming so few calories?*

There is no evidence at all to suggest this possibility.

Actually, most people report improved well-being and much less incidence of the minor infections which prompt visits to the doctor's surgery.

28. *Is there any chance that my skin will be affected by the diet programme?*
Yes . . . in a very positive manner. Micro-Dieters often comment on an improvement in their complexion and skin tone generally. The reason is quite simple: proper nutrition.

29. *What is the role of exercise in your diet plan?*
You will definitely benefit as moderate exercise is certainly important to help your muscle tone. However, do not start a rigorous exercise programme at the same time you start the diet. This will be too much of a strain for your body. Whatever your exercise plan, take it easy at first.

30. *Is it all right to take tranquillisers when I'm dieting?*
There are no *known* contra-indications but if you are taking any kind of prescription whatsoever you are strongly advised to discuss it when you consult your doctor.

31. *Is there any way to get rid of fat faster from specific areas?*
As long as you're drinking just three formula meals a day you will keep losing fat. There is no way of controlling 'target' areas. Various gimmicks and 'devices' have been promoted but have no strong clinical substantiation for their claims.

32. *I've been told that the only way I can really lose 7 extra stone is through surgery. What do you think?*
Try The Micro Diet first. An operation such as gastroplasty, or stomach stapling, should be a 'last resort' treatment. Studies have indicated that Very Low Calorie Diets provide the same success without the very real dangers associated with surgery.

33. *I want to stay on The Micro Diet as my 'sole source' of nutrition for longer than the recommended three weeks. Can I?*

Hospital patients have remained on this kind of formula low-calorie diet for months at a time. However, we insist that three consecutive weeks of 'sole source' be observed, alternated with an 'Add-a-meal' week to help in the re-education of food habits and because each individual is different.

34. *Doesn't this kind of diet cause diarrhoea?*

A small number of people might experience this reaction as a result of the mineral content of the formula. Diluting the diet drink will reduce the problem. If diarrhoea persists for more than two or three days the diet should be temporarily discontinued and your doctor consulted. An allergy to cow's milk could be the culprit, as milk protein is part of the formula.

35. *I suffer from high blood pressure. Is The Micro Diet OK for me?*

A patient's blood pressure is *usually* lowered once they are successfully losing weight with the plan and this is aided by the low sodium content and diuretic effect. Therefore, it is extremely likely that anyone taking anti-hypertensive medication will need the dosage decreased. That's why it's important a physician monitor the situation. The patient should never 'prescribe' for himself.

36. *Is the Very Low Calorie Diet suitable for the elderly?*

For the obese elderly with a medical problem such as maturity onset diabetes, arthritis or high blood pressure, the diet plan, used under medical supervision, could be extremely beneficial. For the overweight elderly without such conditions it is probably unnecessary to lose weight.

37. *Can my overweight 12-year-old son slim with The Micro Diet?*

Growing children should only diet under close medical

86

supervision, but substituting The Micro Diet or Micro Meal food bar for soft drinks, ice cream, chocolate bars etc. will be beneficial for your offspring.

38. *Can a mother use the diet while breast feeding?*

Not as the sole source of nutrition but certainly as a nutritional supplement. The product contains all the vitamins and minerals necessary to promote good health in both mother and child. It might be advisable to mix the formula with milk. A new mother will obviously be medically monitored.

39. *How soon can a new mother, who is not breast feeding, start seriously dieting?*

This is a decision for the doctor although normally a waiting period of two weeks would be sufficient. Mothers who have experienced extreme blood loss or undergone a Caesarian section should probably wait a little longer.

> Lynne Beer of Andover, Hants: 'I lost 23 pounds in the first three weeks. I feel more alive.'

40. *What do I do if I've had my three formula meals and still find that I'm hungry?*

This is really only likely to happen during the first few days on the diet plan. Later, you will not have any cravings at all. To counteract hunger pangs help yourself to an extra serving of the formula. You will be getting much better value from those 110 calories than from any other snack. You really do have to ask yourself *where* you're feeling hungry – your stomach or your head?

41. *Isn't there a danger that I could consume too many vitamins and minerals by having extra formula meals?*

Three drinks of The Micro Diet provide entirely sufficient nutrition for most people's needs. An occasional extra serving is permissible as most vitamins are water soluble and are simply passed through the body if not needed. Supplementary tablets, though, are unnecessary and should not be taken unless recommended by a physician.

42.   *Could I become anaemic on this diet plan?*
There is no evidence whatsoever that anaemia could be a side effect. A woman who suffers heavy and prolonged menstrual periods should bear in mind that a potential for anaemia exists, even when she is not on a weight loss plan.

43.   *Can I give blood while on the rapid weight loss programme?*
Ask the blood bank what their rules are. It's probably not a good idea to give blood while on any kind of weight loss plan because it would reduce your blood volume and could aggravate postural hypotension.

44.   *I usually become terribly depressed when I'm dieting. What do you suggest?*
Most people on The Micro Diet feel exactly the opposite. They tend to become ecstatic as they experience successful weight loss. However, someone who is being treated for severe depression may well find that their physician feels that the stress of a diet plan is too much for them or will want to constantly monitor the situation. Once again, ask your doctor.

45.   *It occurs to me that the liquid-only regime, because it is so low in calories, might make me anorexic. Could this happen?*
Absolutely not. Anorexia Nervosa is a largely misunderstood condition. It is a phobia – a psychological problem. Drastically reducing one's calorie intake as part of a diet plan will not, in itself, lead to Anorexia Nervosa. Further, the anorexic patient particularly shuns carbohydrate which is an integral part of the formula meals and therefore is consumed, three times a day. We do, however, feel strongly that dieters should aim to be

healthy and attractively slim but not thin. Parents of teenage girls should be especially careful to ensure that slimming is towards a realistic goal. A few pounds overweight represents much less of a health hazard than obsessive unnecessary dieting.

46. *I have a tendency towards gout. What do you advise?*
People with gout usually have a higher level of uric acid in their blood. The problem with many diets is that they exacerbate the uric acid level. This would almost certainly occur during the first few days on the diet and medication might be required. Those people who remain on the diet later show a lowered, even normal, uric acid level, and are generally less prone to gout attacks. A doctor's supervision is *vital*.

47. *I know that potassium is important for my heart. Is there really enough in the formula?*
For the normal person who is not taking diuretics (water pills) or other medication, there is sufficient potassium. Clinical studies have not indicated any evidence of potassium depletion. It is imperative that anyone taking medication, particularly for high blood pressure, consult their doctor so that he can monitor the potassium levels and supplement if necessary.

48. *I've had a heart attack and I know I need to lose a lot of weight. Isn't your diet too stressful for me?*
Many heart patients have had positive experience with Very Low Calorie Diets. But we have to emphasise that this is a matter for the judgement of the individual physician – and *constant* monitoring would be necessary. No one with a serious medical condition should embark on any diet programme without the total approval of their doctor. In particular, it's important to mention stroke victims and patients with serious kidney and liver ailments.

49. *What is ketosis and am I likely to get it?*

The incomplete breakdown of fat can leave a residue known as ketone bodies. Ketosis is often caused by high-protein low-carbohydrate diets, i.e. badly balanced diets. The Micro Diet is formulated to give a very specific balance of carbohydrate as well as protein. There is a *moderate* rise in ketone levels in people using a Very Low Calorie Diet which is one reason why the slimmer doesn't feel hungry but does feel well.

50. *I am taking special medication. Is that a problem?*

Repeat: ask your doctor and show him the letter in Appendix B.

51. *I suffer from acute gall bladder attacks. Is it safe to take The Micro Diet?*

Yes. Since Uni-Vite's Micro Diet is a very low-fat diet it would not provoke any gall bladder problems.

52. *Am I too heavy to exercise?*

There's no excuse for not pursuing some kind of mild exercise programme. It doesn't matter how overweight you are, you can always start slowly, spending just a few minutes a day on a non-strenuous routine. Walking is an excellent activity.

53. *I find that I don't need so much sleep when I'm on the 'sole source' plan. Is this usual?*

Quite often slimmers report that they are up and running much earlier in the mornings. Overeating has a definite sedative effect. So dieting itself, balanced nutrition and increased vitality combine to cut the hours of sleep you require. Spend your extra time wisely!

Barbara Harper of Ilminster, Somerset: 'I lost 25 lb. in my first 25 days and now a total of 4 stone. I haven't felt so well in years.'

---

54.   *Does The Micro Diet contain any preservatives?*
There are no preservatives, drugs or diuretics in the formula. It is a natural food supplemented with vitamins, minerals, trace elements and electrolytes.

55.   *What is the shelf life?*
An unopened sachet of the formula is good for 18 months according to Uni-Vite Nutrition.

56.   *Will dieting hurt my sex life?*
On the contrary. Many people enthusiastically comment on a new 'frisky' attitude. It's not surprising really, when you realise the increased physical vigour and mental self-enhancement which accompanies the rapid weight loss.

57.   *I have a sweet tooth. Can I add artificial sweetener to the formula?*
It's entirely up to you. Many people find, however, that they seem to have much less desire for sweet things when consuming Uni-Vite products.

58.   *I've heard of people losing hair on this kind of diet. Can this be true?*
On rare occasions people have reported combing out a few more hairs than normal. There is no cause for alarm. After a very short period of time hair grows normally again. Many more people actually notice the opposite effect – hair growing back. And most people report their nails and hair growing faster.

59.   *I've been told that it's not a good idea to boil the soups. Why is that?*
If you mix the powder with water and then bring to the boil, you will be cooking away some of the vital nutrients, especially vitamins. Always add the powder to hot water, and consume within the next ten minutes or so.

60.   *Should I continue with the diet if I catch the flu?*

It's not advisable to be losing weight while you're sick. Wait until you've recovered.

61.   *I am going through the 'change of life'. Is The Micro Diet OK for me?*
Yes! There's no reason why menopause should hold you back from getting your body in tip-top shape. The diet plan should be a positive step at this stage of your life, making you look and feel better. We have encountered women who have found they experience fewer hot flushes while on the diet.

62.   *The diet doesn't yet seem to have stopped my craving for 'sweets'. Is there anything I can do?*
Take six ½ portions of the formula during the course of the day. After a time most people do report a permanent lessening of their sweet tooth.

63.   *I need to gain weight so I guess your programme is not for me.*
Wrong. By enjoying The Micro Diet formula or Micro Meal bar in addition to normal meals you'll be adding extra protein, vitamins and minerals – particularly when mixed with milk.

64.   *Is it normal to feel so thirsty when I'm dieting?*
Sometimes people are thirsty. It's simply your body's way of telling you that it would like some more fluids to keep it working. Drink more water. It's good for you. In fact, you shouldn't really wait until your body is crying out for water. Liquid is an essential part of the diet plan.

65.   *Is The Micro Diet suitable for vegetarians?*
Yes. For lacto vegetarians not vegans, and for nearly all religious groups. The Chicken & Herb and Beef Soups are the only flavours containing meat extract.

66.   *What about fibre?*
There is no evidence that a diet low in fibre – in the short term – presents any real problem. You can, if you

wish, eat raw high-fibre vegetables or cooked vegetables, e.g. cabbage. There is a full section on fibre in Part II Chapter 1 of this book.

67. *Why is The Micro Diet not sold in chemists?*

Because the advice, support and encouragement of the Advisor is an integral part of the programme.

68. *When I reach my ideal weight I intend to celebrate by going out for a big feast. Is this OK?*

Celebrate with caution. It is not a wise move to suddenly overload your system after it has become used to the 'sole source' regime. Do not eat a large meal after a period on the 330-calorie a day plan. This will be too stressful for your digestive system.

69. *So does every member of the medical profession endorse a 330-calorie a day slimming plan?*

The University of Surrey survey shows that of those G.P.s consulted about the diet, 71% 'actively encouraged' their patients to go on the diet. Less than 5% discouraged patients, presumably on sound medical grounds. Uni-Vite's programme is not a traditional method of slimming. Traditional methods have failed, but as more and more clinical studies on Very Low Calorie Diets find their way into the medical literature, more and more scientists are becoming convinced that this really is the answer.

Those doctors who question VLCDs usually make the following points:

(a) The diet should be medically supervised (we agree – and recommend this).

(b) It's important to teach people better eating habits (that's what half this book is about).

(c) There's a danger of the slimmer losing muscle tissue and protein from vital organs. (The most recent evidence shows the amount of protein lost is no greater than the extra amount of protein gained with the excess weight.)

70. *Why do some people feel cold when they are slimming?*

When people reduce their food intake the body reduces its energy/heat output so unless they wear more clothes (or move to Florida) they will tend to feel the cold.

71. *Does Uni-Vite's Micro Diet contain gluten, making it unsuitable for people with coeliac disease?*

Chocolate, Strawberry, Vanilla, Coffee, Butterscotch and Banana are gluten free. Chicken & Herb and Beef soup do contain gluten.

72. *Are menstrual irregularities a side effect of the diet?*

Occasionally some people do notice menstrual irregularities and this is due to the change in body weight. When the weight stabilises the cycle returns to normal. Some overweight women fail to menstruate, but when they lose weight the periods return.

73. *I sometimes experience leg cramps when I am on the diet. Why is this?*

It is possible that this may arise from losing too much salt from the body. The Micro Diet is relatively low in salt and that may be a contributory factor. If cramp occurs, a little extra salt should be added to the diet.

74. *Why do you lose water when you diet?*

When you diet you obviously reduce your intake of calories. This will mean that initially the body is using up part of its store of glycogen. Since each gram of glycogen in the body binds with four grams of water, when the glycogen is burnt up as energy, it releases four grams of water.

Conversely, when people who have used up their glycogen stores 'binge' on carbohydrate they will notice a rapid weight gain of up to three or four pounds because the glycogen stores are once again filled . . . with both glycogen and water.

75. Why do ex-smokers gain weight?

Because smoking increases your metabolic rate. When they give up smoking the average person will find that their metabolic rate declines by as much as 250 calories a day. That's a lot. If they eat the same as before they will be taking in 3,500 calories more than they need every 14 days.

That will put on 1 lb. per two weeks.

Unless an adjustment is made the pounds will go piling on until they have gained perhaps two stone in the course of a year! And of course the ex-smoker typically turns to chocolate and sweets to console himself – which only compounds the problem. Now smoking is a much bigger health hazard than obesity, so we are very definitely urging you to give up smoking. But we are also urging you to make a specific adjustment in your eating habits at the same time.

76. As there is so much solid evidence behind VLCDs such as The Micro Diet why do the slimming magazines oppose them?

The first thing to remember is that slimming magazines depend for their existence on people anxious to find a solution to the problem of overweight.

The magazines, month in month out, year in year out, publish their latest diets. If any of these diets really worked we presume they would not need to keep inventing new ones! Moreover, most slimming magazines are associated with slimming clubs and these clubs depend for their revenue on people paying the weekly subscription. One club charges over £2.50 per week whether you attend the weigh-in or not and that is about one quarter of the cost of a whole week's Micro Diet food! The slimming clubs and magazines may sincerely believe that people should only lose weight at a 'nice comfortable rate of 1 lb. a week', but we believe such advice is unrealistic. It is a depressingly low rate of weight loss for someone anxious to get rid of their excess fat and it means expensive weekly visits over a much longer period of time. So we wonder whether the opinion on VLCDs as expressed by the slimming magazines can really be as objective as it sounds.

PART II

KEEPING IT OFF

9

RE-EDUCATING YOUR PALATE

There is no question that many people have a natural tendency to gain weight easily.

But there is no avoiding the fact that over-eating – even acknowledging that that is a relative term, not necessarily a criticism – is the cause of overweight. A person who only needs 1,200 calories of food energy a day is overeating on a 1,500 calorie intake – even though 1,500 calories is relatively low compared with the average person's energy needs.

If you fall into this category, it is undoubtedly unfair; but now that you *have* lost your excess fat, having failed so many times before, you can switch your priority to maintaining your new trimmer physique. Through following The Micro Diet you will have been able to estimate just how many calories you can safely consume without rolls of fat appearing. Most Micro-Dieters, therefore, continue using the formula meals to replace one meal a day or 'sole source' one day a week when it is a convenient part of their lifestyle.

But the prime aim of this section of the book is to make you aware of other changes you can make in your everyday eating habits.

So why do you eat?

Do you eat to live or live to eat? Some people view food emotionally. They eat for all sorts of reasons other than simple hunger. Boredom, worry, stress, habit, impulse. We eat for 'mind' reasons as well as 'body' reasons.

It is important to view food in its proper perspective: to

be enjoyed, relished, something absolutely necessary, of course, but not something to dominate our thoughts or be an emotional crutch. Think carefully about these questions and answer them honestly and fully:

Do you ever eat to reward yourself?

You worked hard today, coped especially well with the children, helped a friend, so you ate something special.

Do you always finish everything on your plate?

It is immoral to waste food. Right? Scandalous when there are starving children in the Third World. Right? Wrong! It is illogical to overburden your body with more than you need and the starving children would be better off with a donation to a suitable charity.

Do you eat absent-mindedly?

Do you pick at leftovers while talking? Munch snacks while watching TV? One of the best examples of 'mindless calories' is when you visit the pictures. You buy a box of popcorn or a packet of chocolate. The first two mouthfuls are delicious. Then you go on 'automatic pilot'. Your hand keeps dipping into the box and finding its own way towards your mouth. The next thing you know is that there are none left and you never even noticed they were going down. Pure mindless calories!

Do you eat because you're bored?

There's not much to do. You're alone. So you make yourself something to eat. Everybody does it but some of us do it a lot too often.

Do you eat when you're worried?

Everybody gets tense and anxious. Nervous under pressure. So you eat. You're a little unsure of yourself at a social occasion. So you eat. It's something to do with your hands. Funny, because that's exactly what smokers say . . . only they use tobacco to calm their nerves. Eating because you are worried may well seem a 'natural reaction' to you but it's not very logical. Eating is hardly going to make the problem go away. In fact, you may well end up with two problems: the original one *and* being overweight.

Do you eat because it is lunchtime?

Many people eat simply because of the time of day. It's 8 a.m. so breakfast is required. At 1 p.m. it is time to take a break from work and go to the pub. Or it is 6 p.m. and the family are all at home for dinner. You might not be hungry but the eating routine has to be kept.

Do you eat to be polite?

You're attending a business lunch and don't feel you should risk abusing your host's hospitality? Your friend wants you to sample the cake she has just baked? You don't have to do it! If you explain that you have to watch your shape they will understand.

These are just a few reasons why we eat. Some of them were physical but many of them were really feeding your mind. It's your body, however, that picked up the extra calories.

Do you know how big your stomach is? Make a fist and look at it. That's how little food it takes to fill your stomach.

If you feel that you, too, may eat for reasons other than nutrition, answer just a few more questions and then we can start on ways to deal with the issue.

1. Think back to when you first noticeably put on weight. What was your age? Your financial situation? How were your relationships – with your parents, your friends, the opposite sex?
2. What did your answers to the above questions tell you about yourself?

They probably brought home to you how often you (and lots of other people) eat for reasons quite unconnected with being hungry. The chances are that some of your eating is really a reflex action. Unthinking. If you need to keep your weight under control you can't afford to indulge in calories you don't fully enjoy.

Here's a project that's fun and will be a revelation! At the next convenient weekend (so you have time) make a favourite meal. Try and ensure that it includes a really tasty meat or fish dish and your favourite vegetables, plus a good choice of fresh fruit and some cheese. Include a luscious dessert.

Now spread it all on the table before you start. Pick up the plate, look carefully at each piece of food. Take up a piece on your fork. Smell it. Savour it. Now chew it carefully and concentrate on the taste and the texture. Did you know that food tastes different depending on whether it touches the front or back of your tongue?

Now do the same for every different type of food on your plate. Notice which you liked most.

Have another 'round' eating slowly and savouring the food. Stop and consider how hungry you are. Continue and stop frequently to consider the same question. 'Are you still hungry?' When you have reached the point that you can sense that you're no longer hungry – simply stop eating.

Perhaps for the first time in a long while, you will have really concentrated on your food, appreciated it, sensed its effect. It should have been a sensually pleasurable experience – rather than the rushed grab we so often make our eating occasions. And what do you do with any food left when you have stopped? Throw it away. After you've done that, notice how you felt. About the meal and about throwing the leftovers away.

'Calorie counting'

This book could not have been written without frequent use of the word 'calorie'. It's an irreplaceable part of the vocabulary of every diet-conscious person. But do you really know what a calorie is? You should; and equally you should be aware of the varying values of what you can get nutritionally to make calories count rather than simply counting calories.

A calorie is the measurement of the potential energy in food. It is the amount of energy (heat) required to raise the temperature of 1 kilogram of water by 1 degree C. The average hourly calorie output of 12 people is equivalent to a one-bar electric fire!

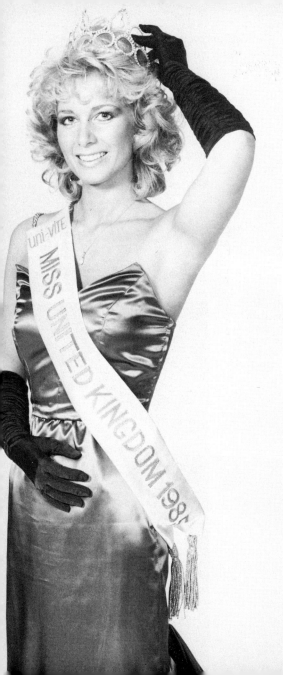

Lovely Mandy
Shires lost
an amazing
28lb in
28 days –
and went on
to the Miss
U.K. title!

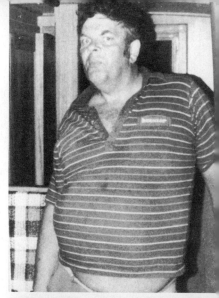

Slim and trim now,
Cornish businessman
John Bray melted away
seven stone in as many
months winning himself
the title of Micro–Dieter
of the Year.

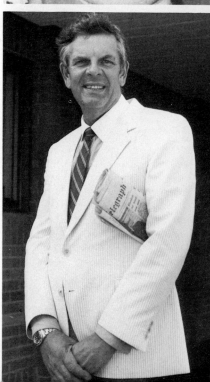

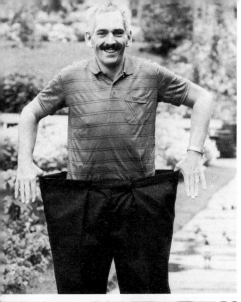

Smiling in the rain, Manchester's Ray Berry filled these massive pants just seven months earlier. Ray has lost ten stone.

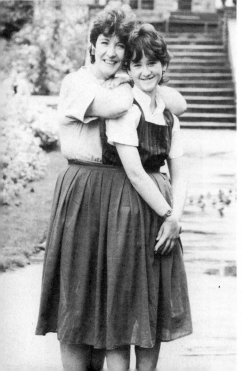

North Wales mum, Shirley Wynne comfortably shares her once tight skirt with 15 year old daughter Tracie. Tracie weighs less than the weight Shirley shed.

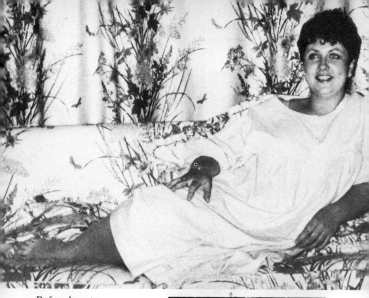

Before beauty consultant Joanne Butler (above: taking the weight off her feet) lost a staggering four stone, she would never have contemplated wearing these stripes.

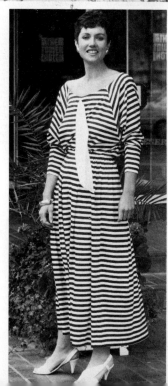

Now, although we believe the counting of every last calorie in our food is boring, unnecessary and part of 'old style' dieting, we certainly appreciate that you can't ignore the effects of calories. So a more interesting way of dramatising the energy differences of food to enable you to make more sensible choices is to see how much of various types of food would equal 110 calories – the same as *one* serving of The Micro Diet containing all those nutrients!

Visualising 110 calories – This is what you get for 110 calories.

6 teaspoons sugar
1 tablespoon mayonnaise
22 peanuts
2 thin rashers streaky bacon
3 sardines
3 plain biscuits
¼ of a small pork pie
100 g/4 oz. grilled white fish
3 tablespoons sweet pickle
½ pint beer
1 measure gin and 1 small bottle tonic
1 small glass wine
1 small glass milk
50 g/2 oz. ice cream
1 small currant bun
3 level teaspoons butter
1 fried egg (medium)
3 oz. boiled rice
1 small doughnut
2 small slices wholemeal bread
1 small 'Kit-Kat'
2 slices corned beef
4½ oz. baked potato
1 oz. fresh coconut
2 fudge sweets (1 oz.)
3 level teaspoons flour

2 thin slices lean ham
3 thin slices lean roast beef
2 slices chicken breast
145 g/5 oz. baked beans
1 carton flavoured yoghurt
1 cube edam cheese (1" cube)
4 slices Ryvita
1 cup breakfast cereal without milk
1 finger of shortbread
1 large banana
2 tablespoons whipping cream
1 small sausage
1 tube polo mints
2 baked fish fingers
1 small carton cottage cheese
2 oz. fried mushrooms
½ large corn-on-the-cob
3½ oz. can tuna in brine
3 'After Eight' mints
½ pt. unsweetened orange juice
3½ oz. boiled prawns
1 can orangeade
3 thin slices garlic sausage

Don't count calories – make every calorie count!

Case history

Name: Muri Symons
Home town: St Helier
Weight loss: 2 st. 7 lb.

Cruise ship pianist Muri Symons couldn't resist the
mountains of food served up while entertaining on
the ocean waves.

Back home in Jersey, with her evening dresses
bursting at the seams, she felt 'miserable, heavy and
old' until she lost 2½ stone in less than three
months.

'Even though I'm in my fifties, I cannot remember
feeling so well since I was a teenager,' says Muri.
'I've lost inches from my waist, my arthritis pains
have halved and my hiatus hernia stopped bothering
me. Last year I shuffled with great difficulty – now I
can actually run again.'

'Hidden' Calories

We have emphasised that we don't believe in endless
calorie counting. But it doesn't mean that you can ignore
the calories or the calorific value of certain foods. If you
know the type of food to treat with great caution, you do
not have to bother counting calories in the sort of food
that, in practice, you won't overeat.

So the concept of 'hidden calories' is useful. They are
the foods that are surprisingly calorific. Here are just a
few of those surprises!

Salad dressing (250 calories extra)
Salads can be unlimited, right? Yes – but salad dressing
certainly can't. Just 2 oz. casually poured on is about 250
calories.

Sour cream (60 calories extra)

A baked potato is an ideal food. The sour cream on it probably costs at least 60 calories.

Biscuits (150 calories extra)

A mid-morning break with three chocolate biscuits. The biscuits alone cost 150 calories – that's equivalent to ¾ hour of brisk walking. Worth it? The choice is yours.

Grilled fish with butter (110 calories extra)

The grilled fish was a great decision – the ½ oz. butter added 100 casual, hidden calories.

A ham sandwich (315 calories)

A single ham sandwich will be 315 calories. Bit of a surprise.

Peaches and cream (200 calories)

The average portion will 'set you back' 200 calories because all canned fruit has TWICE the calories of fresh fruit and cream is very concentrated calories.

1 Mars bar (320 calories)

2 oz. of chocolate will give you a quick energy fix – but an hour later it leaves you feeling hungry. It's all too easy to eat a bar of chocolate, for example, while driving the car. 320 mindless calories!

A glass of wine (100 calories)

2 glasses of wine are 200 calories. Fine as long as you 'trade' them for some exercise.

A pint of beer (190 calories)

A couple of 'swift pints' – 380 calories. If you did that every night it is the same as adding a whole day's extra food onto each 7-day week!

A 'little pork pie' (270 calories)

Some snacks are just loaded with hidden calories.

Peanut butter (35 calories)

Just one teaspoon is 35 calories so think again before having a taste or liberally spreading on bread!

Bacardi and coke (125 calories)

A measure of rum is one thing – 50 calories. Mix it with a small bottle of coke and you're adding another 75 calories. Go for the diet version.

Quiche (585 calories)

What about this one? We think of a slice of quiche as a healthy, nourishing food. But an average slice of 5 oz./150g costs 585 calories. Beware!

Avocado pear (235 calories)

Just half an appetising avocado!

Let's be clear. It doesn't mean you can't have any of the above. It does mean you shouldn't mislead yourself by ignoring the 'hidden calories'. Being aware of these hidden calories in the 'extras' is half the battle. For instance, think back to the last time you went to a self-service motorway cafe. Do you know what they normally put first in the range, as you start sliding your tray down the counter? Desserts, cream cakes, ice cream. Because restaurateurs know that when you're hungry you'll want to grab precisely that type of food.

Here is a suggestion for when you are next in a self-service cafe. Buy the main course – for example, meat or fish. Then, when you've eaten that, ask yourself: 'Do I *really* want dessert?' You'll notice a big difference in your attitude. Firstly, there's all the bother of queueing all over again. Secondly, you are now questioning whether you want dessert, after you already have begun to feel full. So now if you really want the dessert it is a conscious decision – not an unthinking grab for food at the very moment you are likely to make the worst choice of food, i e. when you are hungry!

The easy changes

Preparing food becomes after a time, a matter of habit. Yet it's quite possible to eliminate an amazing number of calories by really simple changes. The point about these changes is that, individually, they don't seem to amount to much over the course of even a month. Yet, over a year, each one can make a real impact, and several changes together will accumulate to a dramatic effect.

Here is a list of some easy changes you can make. Your body is not like an adding (or subtracting) machine, so you can't assume that just because you cut out, for example, four teaspoonfuls of sugar a day, you will automatically lose 12 lb. a year. The relationship, in practice, between calories and weight loss is not that simple, but the list indicates the exciting potential.

Case history

Name: Margaret Crellin
Home town: Egremont
Weight loss: 1 st. 7 lb.

Margaret Crellin's 1½-stone weight loss is more meaningful to her than someone else's 6-stone success.

For Margaret, 45, suffers from a rare muscle wasting disease and finds she is much more mobile.

'I feel so much stronger. I can spend more time on my feet and out of the wheelchair,' she enthuses. 'I'm less dependent on others and that's the greatest bonus of all.'

Margaret felt so well, in fact, that she even managed a gruelling 350-mile charity wheelchair push from her home in Egremont, Cumbria, to London. Now she is continuing to use The Micro Diet as part of her weight maintenance.

The Easy Changes

What you may do now	What you could do	What it would save each time	What it would save in a year (calories)	How many lb. less it could be
1 spoon of sugar per cup of tea or coffee (say 4 cups per day)	Use sweetener or stop using sugar	20 cal. per teaspn. i.e. 80 cal. per day	29,200	8½ lb.
5 pints of beer a week	Make just three occasions a half i.e. drink 3½ pts.	273 cals. per week	14,200	4 lb.
Snack 1 packet (2oz.) peanuts whilst watching TV (twice a week)	Only eat at the table therefore NO TV snacks	324 cals. per packet, 648 cals. per week	33,700	10 lb.
Drink gin & tonic (4 drinks a week)	Switch to low-calorie tonic	40 cals. per drink, 160 cals. per week	8,320	2½ lb.
2 fried rashers of bacon (twice a week)	Grill the bacon	75 cals. per week	3,900	1 lb.
4 fried sausages a week	Grill the sausages and prick them to let the fat run out	44 cals. per week	2,290	½ lb.
4 fried eggs each week	Fry in a non-stick pan without fat or oil	20 cals. per egg, 80 cals. per week	4,160	1 lb.
You thicken your gravy with 1 oz. of flour	Don't thicken the gravy	100 cals. per time, 200 cals. per week	10,400	3 lb.

You use 5 oz. full cream milk on your cornflakes (3 times a week)	Use a little less skimmed milk (3 oz.)	65 cals. per serving, 195 cals. per week	10,140	3 lb.
You have 2 slices of toast and marmalade using ½ oz. of butter per slice (twice a week) (That's 430 cals. per sitting)	Take 1½ slices of toast, use low-calorie margarine (hardly noticeable with the marmalade on top) spread the marmalade thinner – the taste is strong enough. The new total is 200 cal. per serving.	140 cals. i.e. 280 per week	14,560	4 lb.
You have a bowl of Cream of Tomato soup 6 oz.	You have a bowl of low-calorie soup	69 cals.	3,590	1 lb.
You have a fried fish and chip supper once a week. Av. is 6 oz. of fish and say 6 oz. chips. 6 oz. chips = 435 cals. 6 oz. cod in batter = 340 cals. } 775	You grill 6 oz. of cod and fry 4 oz. of large chips. Small chips soak up more oil because there are more of them and the area covered by the oil is much greater. New total is: Fish 130 cals. Chips 290 cals. 420 cals.	335 cals. per week	17,420	5 lb.

You have apple pie and 2 oz. cream	You splash out on half the cream i.e. 1 oz.	125 cals.	6,500	2 lb.
You use 2 tablespoons of cooking oil in the frying pan/casserole to brown the meat before preparing goulash/stew	You cut this to ¾ tablespoonful	158 cals. (say twice a week)	16,430	5 lb.

Further Easy Changes

You use mayonnaise for Prawn Cocktail	You mix one third mayonnaise with two thirds yoghurt	67 cals. per portion
You make a beef strogonoff using 5 oz. soured cream	You use 3 oz. natural yoghurt	65 cals. per portion
You use cream in raspberry fool	You use yoghurt instead	180 cals. per portion
You make a tomato salad adding vinaigrette dressing instead	You use lemon juice instead	145 cals. average per person per serving

Salad dressings use a high proportion of oil which is very, very calorific. Use yoghurt or lemon juice. The true taste of the salad is better preserved.

We hope more examples are superfluous. There is no food that is truly 'off limits'. But by making sensible substitutes, easy changes, you can effect savings that over the course of a year have an incredible impact. Re-read the list and think about it.

What did you do? You . . .

1. Cut out sugar in tea and coffee. It really can be done in a couple of weeks. You'll hate the taste the first day. Persevere and by the end of the second week you'll probably hate the taste of sugar.

2. You drank just a little less beer, but made the same number of pub visits.

3. You used low-calorie mixers, squashes and soft drinks.

4. You grilled your food instead of frying it.

5. You didn't thicken your gravy or sauces with flour.

6. You used skimmed milk.

7. You ate a little less toast. You used low-calorie margarine and spread the marmalade/jam just enough to taste.

8. You used low-calorie soup not cream of soup.

9. You ate a little less cream – and you substituted yoghurt for cream and mayonnaise.

10. You used lemon juice instead of vinaigrette or oil dressing.

None of the above were exactly traumatic changes were they? You are still eating the same kind of food. But the accumulative effect over the course of a year could be a saving of 100,000 calories! You've potentially saved 28 lb. or 2 stone compared with the result of continuing the old habits.

See how a few cooking changes can help you maintain your weight? See how much margin for error you have by making the easy changes?

And remember that as a 'safety net' you have always the opportunity to go on The Micro Diet 'sole source' for a day or two.

Now let's look at 'the big picture'. Observing the easy changes can certainly make an excellent contribution to your overall diet.

But nutritionists today are recommending some fundamental changes to the nation's eating habits as the benefits of certain foods and the hazards of others become more and more apparent.

Let's look at two of the key subjects under scrutiny – fibre and fat.

The fibre factor

There has been much debate in the last few years about the need for adequate dietary fibre. The experts who have conducted trials with VLCDs firmly believe that there is no harmful effect from a short-term lack of fibre during rapid weight loss.

However, the evidence is growing that a long-term lack of fibre is a major contributory factor in the development of large bowel disease, including irritable bowel syndrome, constipation, diverticulitis and colon cancer . . . the second most common cancer which, in fact, accounted for 12.7% of the deaths from all tumours in 1980 in England and Wales. A high percentage of all Britons over the age of 40 years have some problems with obstructions in the colon. The British Medical Journal has reported that 62 out of 70 patients experienced relief when they ate a high-fibre diet.

The Royal College of Physicians of London has recommended that more fibre be included in the British diet and their position was recently strongly endorsed by the NACNE report. Discussing the optimum level, the NACNE report states: 'Dietary fibre intakes of 30 grams or more are associated with a lower prevalance of diverticular disease in vegetarians and are used with beneficial effect in the treatment of constipation and diverticular disease.'

Fibre consumption in Britain today is low: an average of just 20 grams per day whereas intakes of 50–120 grams per day are estimated for Africans living in rural communities. In Britain during the war, says the report, 32–40 grams was the average intake. At present, UK vegetarians consume, on average, 42 grams of fibre a day.

Looking ahead over the next 15 years, the experts would like to see the average British intake increase to 30 grams a day with cereal fibre, in particular, being included because it is more effective in increasing faecal weight than fruit or vegetable fibre. In the short term they strongly recommend a move towards 23 grams per head per day.

The Uni-Vite Micro Meal contains 8 grams per bar – a third of the NACNE recommendations.

But can fibre help weight control?

There is evidence that it can. Dr K. W. Heaton, writing in the *Lancet*, showed that eating high-fibre bread as opposed to white bread enabled the body to pass some calories through the system without being absorbed and to speed that transit by five times or more. His research sparked additional studies at the Department of Food Science and Human Nutrition at Michigan State University. This showed that people on a high-fibre diet voluntarily ate less and appeared to absorb less fat in addition to the weight loss effect owing to calories being 'passed through' the body. Their report stimulated headlines in the USA claiming: 'The more bread you eat the more weight you lose.'

The evidence for inclusion of adequate dietary fibre is persuasive as part of a long-term weight maintenance programme, but like everything else in life there needs to be a balance. Too much fibre causes the body to fail to absorb some essential minerals, especially zinc.

So how to obtain sufficient fibre in ordinary food? Listed here are some of the most common sources (fibre itself isn't calorific but the foods that contain it are).

	Amount to produce 23 grams of dietary fibre		Calories involved
Unprocessed bran	52 g	(1.8 oz.)	107
All Bran	86 g	(3 oz.)	235
Dried Apricots	96 g	(3.4 oz.)	175
Beans (baked)	315 g	(11.1 oz.)	202
Wholemeal bread	271 g	(9.5 oz.)	585
Carrots	793 g	(27.8 oz.)	182
Blackcurrants	264 g	(9.3 oz.)	74

In practice, of course, you would be eating a mixture of foods to provide enough fibre and you can probably rely on your current diet to provide at least half of what you need, especially if you are eating from the above list.

By studying the above plan you can devise your own low-calorie/high-fibre plan. Try to include foods that contain fibre.

Alternatively, you can add plain bran to breakfast cereal, yoghurt or hamburgers or, of course, one of your glasses of The Micro Diet.

The fat factor

Generally, we would be better off reducing saturated fats – that's animal fat and dairy fat. Unsaturated fats, which include most vegetable oils (except coconut and palm oil) raise cholesterol levels to a lesser extent and this is now generally considered a more beneficial form in which to take fat, either in cooking oil or as a spread. Do check labels to make sure the fat is indeed unsaturated. Sunflower oil has the highest percentage of polyunsaturated fatty acids. Ounce for ounce, of course, all types of fat are equally calorific.

The link between coronary heart disease and dietary fat is well established. Death rates for coronary heart disease in the UK are among the highest in the world. In England and Wales in 1980, males *under the age of 65* accounted for 31% of deaths from coronary artery disease. There is now a strong concensus of opinion that a reduction of total fat in the diet to 30–35% of total energy or calorie intake is needed to combat the menace, with saturated fatty acid intake providing an average of 10%.

The latest report on the subject produced by the National Advisory Committee on Nutrition Education (NACNE), came to the conclusion that an immediate aim for the 1980s should be a) Reduction of the average total fat intake by 10% from 128 g (38% of total energy kcal) to the new figure of 115 g (34% of total kcal); b) Reduction of average saturated fatty acids intake from 59 g (18% of

Case history

Name: Christine Penney
Home town: Poole
Weight loss: 4 stone

Community nurse Christine Penney is in better shape now than she was on her wedding day 22 years ago.

Chris, of Poole, Dorset, has lost more than four stone – the first stone slipped away in less than three weeks.

Needless to say she's thrilled with her success. 'I'd struggled to lose weight on other diets and the weight I lost soon reappeared. The four stone I've lost with The Micro Diet I've kept off for 10 months.'

Like so many women, Chris's weight problems became worse with the birth of each successive child – three in total – until she reached a peak of 13 stone 6 lb.

After her first three weeks of 'sole source', Chris took one week's break, adding low-calorie meals. She continued on her weight loss path by going 'sole source' during the week and having conventional meals at the weekend with her family.

Now 5′ 2″-tall Chris, a trim 9 st. 6 lb., says: 'I'd stopped going to keep-fit classes because I was acutely embarrassed heaving my leotard over my rolls of fat. I'll never get that way again! . . . I feel better than I've ever felt before – I feel fantastic!'

total energy) to 50 g (15% of total) i.e. a 15% reduction. Put into the context of the daily diet of an average Englishwoman, she would be advised to limit her fat intake to a maximum of 3 ounces (that, of course, includes fat from all sources i.e. in milk, meat, chocolate, etc., as well as the 'obvious' form of fat which is butter or margarine).

Creating your own balance

A major advantage of the Uni-Vite meal plans is that a day's supply already includes an ideal balance of protein, carbohydrate and fat, plus all the vitamins and minerals you need, during weight loss. Ordinary calorie tables can be boring and basically unnecessary. So in their place we are listing some foods we commonly consume so that, at a glance, you can see whether they contribute mainly protein, carbohydrate or fat or whether they are unexpectedly calorific. This unique chart allows you to appreciate why you should concentrate on some foods and be wary of others.

Food	Protein content	Carbohydrate content	Fat content	Calories per oz.
Lard	0	0	99%	254
Margarine	0	0	81%	208
Butter	0	0	82%	211
Double cream	2%	2%	48%	127
Low-fat spread	0	0	41%	104
Bacon (grilled)	25%	0	36%	120
Luncheon meat	13%	6%	27%	89
Pork sausage	11%	10%	32%	105
Almonds	17%	4%	54%	161
Cheddar cheese	26%	0	34%	116
Roast peanuts	24%	9%	49%	162
Roast lamb	20%	0	26%	90
Eggs	12%	0	11%	42
Ham	18%	0	5%	34
Potato crisps	6%	49%	36%	152
Sardines in oil	24%	0	14%	62
Milk chocolate	8%	59%	30%	151
Liver (fried)	27%	7%	13%	72
Milk	3%	5%	4%	19
Cottage cheese	14%	1%	4%	27
Chocolate biscuits	6%	67%	28%	149
Stewing steak	31%	0	11%	64
Ice cream	4%	25%	7%	48
Potato (fried)	4%	37%	11%	72

Fried fish in batter	20%	8%	10%	57
Jam tarts	4%	63%	15%	109
Roast chicken	25%	0	5%	42
Low fat yoghurt (fruit)	5%	18%	1%	27
Grilled fish (white)	21%	0	1%	27
Brown bread	9%	45%	2%	64
White bread	8%	50%	2%	66
Crispbread (rye)	9%	71%	2%	91
Cornflakes	9%	85%	2%	105
Spaghetti	14%	84%	1%	108
Skimmed milk	3%	5%	0	9
Baked beans	5%	10%	0	18
Honey	1%	74%	5%	82
Spirits	0	0	0	63
White wine (dry)	0	1%	0	19
Apples	0	12%	0	13
Potatoes (boiled)	1%	20%	0	23
Peas (boiled)	5%	8%	0	15
Brussel sprouts (boiled)	3%	2%	0	5
Spinach (boiled)	5%	1%	0	9
Unsweetened orange juice	1%	9%	0	11
Beer	0	2	0	9
Black pudding (fried)	13	15	22	89
Pork pie	10	25	27	107
Jam	1	69	0	74
Avocado pear	4	2	22	64
Custard sauce (made with powder)	4	17	4	34
Rice	7	87	1	103
Digestive biscuits	10	66	21	134
Doughnuts	6	49	16	99
Scotch egg	12	12	21	80
Vegetable oil	0	0	99	256
Minced beef	19	0	16	63
Canned tuna (in oil)	23	0	22	82
Scampi (fried)	12	29	18	90
Onions (fried)	2	10	33	98
Raisins	1	64	0	70
Peanut butter	23	13	54	178

Drinking chocolate powder	6	77	6	104
Coca-cola	0	11	0	11
Sherry	0	4	0	34
Cream of tomato soup (canned)	1	6	3	16
Cream cheese	3	0	47	125
Bananas	1	19	0	23
Cream crackers	10	68	16	125
Sweetcorn	3	16	1	22
Coconut (fresh)	3	4	36	100
Toffees (mixed)	2	71	17	123
Mandarin oranges (canned)	1	14	0	16
Sausage roll (flaky pastry)	7	33	36	137
Fish fingers	14	17	13	66
Muesli	13	66	8	105
Meringues	5	95	0	108
Chocolate eclairs	4	38	24	107
Beefburgers (fried)	20	7	17	75
Jelly (made with water)	1	14	0	17
Madeira cake	5	58	17	112
Roast potatoes	3	27	5	45
Broad beans (boiled)	4	7	1	14
Scrambled egg	11	0	23	70
Ribena (undiluted)	0	61	0	65
French dressing	0	0	73	187
Mayonnaise	2	0	79	205
Spaghetti (canned in tomato sauce)	2	12	0	17
Grilled steak	27	0	12	62
Roast pork	27	0	20	82

Percentage calculated on weight basis

Hazel Thompson devoted two pages of the *Townswoman*, the national magazine of the Townswomen's Guild, to her Micro Diet experience under the heading: 'The final solution, or how I lost a stone and gained my sanity.'

Hazel, who admitted to being 'very sceptical' when she started the diet, was thrilled with her success and even escaped unscathed from an 'accidental trip' to Harrods Food Hall and an evening helping out in a friend's restaurant.

She was impressed too, with the attention she received from her Advisor, writing: 'Another valuable service is provided – each slimmer is allocated an Advisor, whom they can ring up at any time with any problem or query. If, for instance, you have a burning desire for a bag of chips and feel you're about to succumb, ring your Advisor and he or she will "talk you through it" . . . rather like AA. The Advisors have all used the product and are thoroughly familiar with every aspect of it.'

119

10

CHANGING YOUR HABITS

The easy changes were really common sense. In fact, we recommend you write out the main suggestions and hang them up in the kitchen. Since habits die hard, we all need a reminder.

Habits are not something we often consciously form, but to change them does require conscious effort. Now the reasons you were overeating – compared with your personal metabolic needs – was because you just didn't realise that your body needed fewer calories and because you were operating on 'automatic pilot'. Your job is to 'programme' that automatic pilot with a different set of instructions.

Recognising the problem

The best possible way to be conscious of your current habits is quite simply to take two pieces of paper. On one piece of paper write down *everything* you eat tomorrow. 'Everything' means exactly that – meals, snacks, tasting food which you are cooking, titbits, and don't forget milk and sugar in tea or coffee.

You must also record what you were doing at the time – standing by the fridge, watching TV, reading, sitting at the table. Then do the same for the next day. It honestly will not take more than five minutes a day.

What it will do is surprise you. We're quite sure you will be staggered at the number of occasions you eat other than sitting at your table. It's a safe bet that you also find yourself eating for other reasons than hunger. You may be surprised, too, when you remember your mood while you were eating. Were you fed up, worried, bored? That's significant, isn't it?

WHEN YOU SHOP, USE A LIST AND STICK TO IT. SHOP AS SOON AS POSSIBLE AFTER A MEAL.

___

It is a positive fact that people make more sensible food choices and purchase less calorific food when they are not hungry. We are all suggestable.

Please don't just acknowledge this advice – practice it. Plan your next shopping trip after lunch, for instance, and you'll be amazed at the difference.

Always have three meals a day

To keep your body satisfied it is important to eat regularly. Breakfast should not be skipped, but, of course, many of us feel we simply 'can't face anything' first thing in the morning or we 'just don't have time'. The ideal solution is The Micro Diet.

In one glass, in one minute, you mix one-third of your day's nutritional requirements. What a great start to the day! Lunch and dinner also have their part to play because, by taking proper nourishment at regular mealtimes, you may dispel the urge to snack in between meals.

Don't eat too late

'Breakfast is the most important meal of the day. Don't eat immediately before going to bed.'

Common enough advice – and certainly sound advice, for the slimmer, but do you know why?

Meals taken early in the day have the effect of inducing peaks of hormonal activity in a way that fights fat. Conversely, if you eat late, the lower hormone levels essentially reduce the body's natural ability to metabolise fat.

121

The practical result is astonishing. Scientists at the University of Minnesota actually prepared a paper entitled: 'We are not only *what* we eat – but *when* we eat'.

They reached this conclusion after a highly imaginative series of experiments in which one group of people were given a precisely measured 2,000-calorie a day menu. They were instructed to eat only breakfast. The other group ate only dinner – but the same 2,000 calories. The 'early eating' group lost an average of 1½ lb. a week, while the 'late meals' group *gained* about 1 lb. a week.

Then the groups changed over. The early eaters began consuming their calories late in the day; the former late eaters became the breakfast brigade. Again the early eaters lost weight and the late eaters gained. These results were confirmed in a study conducted for the US Government at Natick, Massachussetts, where the direct effect of eating early in the day rather than later was 1 lb. a week weight loss.

While we are obviously not proposing to cut out the evening meal – the main social meal in the way we order a modern life – it is clearly only common sense to ensure that we enjoy adequate breakfast and lunch and to be careful when evening arrives.

ALWAYS EAT SITTING DOWN AND ALWAYS EAT IN A SPECIFIC EATING PLACE!

Eating should be something you concentrate on and thoroughly enjoy. The Uni-Vite philosophy is that food is great, and eating is one of life's major pleasures. But be a gourmet – not a gourmand.

'Gourmet' means someone who loves food, and is interested in taste. A 'gourmand' is someone who eats a lot – for the sake of eating. A glutton.

People who really love food savour the flavour. You don't have to eat 10 oz. of steak to get the taste of steak. 6 oz. eaten slowly with relish, will taste just as good. If you've ever been in a top French restaurant in France you'll discover two things. The food is exquisite, and the helpings are much smaller than would be served in the UK. They are gourmets – not gourmands.

The same is true of the Japanese. They eat lots of courses but each one is a small delicacy. You feast but you don't feel full. It's a relief to get up from the table and not feel overstuffed. You feel good.

The English Royal Family is probably involved in more social eating with more rich food at more lavish banquets than anyone. They eat some of each dish – quite deliberately leaving some so they are 'ready' for the next course. This way everything can be tasted and enjoyed.

So, if you respect food you will make eating an occasion. You can't concentrate on the taste if you are reading or watching TV or doing a crossword. You have no appreciation of how much you eat or its quality. The same is true about eating standing up. 'Grabbing something to eat' as you walk past the fridge is not respecting food.

If you sit down in one place you will learn to feel the effect of food, learn to eat for taste and not out of boredom. You will also be in a position to sense when you no longer feel hungry. If you mindlessly grab handfuls of peanuts, crisps or chocolate whilst watching TV, you have no chance of registering whether you're hungry or not. Eat in one place. Eat sitting down and concentrate ONLY on eating. Avoid 'mindless calories'.

Practise leaving something on your plate

Now this will be a little harder to swallow! At the beginning of the programme please make a conscious decision to leave something on your plate. There is really good reason for this.

We are trained to eat too much! We start with a natural instinct to stop eating when we are no longer hungry – but this instinct is suppressed. A baby that is breast fed will eat as much as it needs. Like an animal in the wild it instinctively stops eating when it is satisfied. When the baby is switched to a bottle the mother can now see if anything is left, and the reaction of most mothers is to encourage the baby to finish it up – even if left to himself the child would have stopped feeding. Statistically, bottle fed babies are heavier than breast fed babies.

So begins the habit of finishing up everything on the plate, 'because it's a waste not to'.

When you leave something on your plate you are saying two things to your subconscious. First, you are saying that you have control, you do not need to eat just because it's there.

Secondly, and far more importantly, it reduces your emotional and psychological dependence on food. The first time you deliberately leave something you'll probably feel guilty – for all the reasons we've said. But do it. Do it at each evening meal for a week and you'll discover a new feeling. You'll no longer feel uneasy at leaving food – you'll feel in control. The beneficial effect on your subconscious attitude to food will be immense.

Don't pass this advice over as a 'fad' piece of psychology – it really works.

Eat slowly

If you eat slowly you will find that it may take as few as 12 bites of food to satisfy your hunger. Try it! Observe how you feel. You'll find that the desire to continue eating after the first dozen mouthfuls is mostly for taste – or for social reasons.

All this is part of the general encouragement to listen to your body. If you are aware of it, in tune with it, you'll gradually get back to the condition you were born with, the ability to eat what you really need, when you really need it. Eating slowly and stopping when you've had enough. When you're eating just stop every now and then, and ask yourself, 'Am I still hungry?' If not – STOP.

Cut down on sugar

Yes, that's very common advice – but here's why.

Sugar has no other form of nutrition but calories. 'Empty calories' is a good phrase. It's absolutely valueless for anything but sweetening and energy.

You can learn to hate it in tea or coffee. Ask anyone who has given it up. It actually tastes awful if they accidently drink a cup that has been sweetened. By far the best way is to cut down by half for a week, then half again for another week and by the end of the third week eliminate it altogether. You really can do it.

Whilst it is (comparatively) easy to eliminate sugar from your tea and coffee (and thereby potentially save over 40,000 calories a year!), reducing sugar in other ways requires some vigilance. Reading labels on cans and bottles is instructive. An easy way to cut out totally unnecessary calories is never to buy canned fruit in syrup. A less obvious way is to reduce on additions like tomato sauce, which have a high sugar content.

Make your natural laziness work for you!

It is obvious that you can't eat what is not available! One Uni-Vite Advisor we know, keeps no chocolate or sweets in the house at all. If she wants them she has to go out to the local shops. So she asks herself the key question. 'I can have it if I want it, but do I really want it?' Mostly she doesn't.

On a more everyday basis: if you are making toast – put one slice in the toaster at a time. If you make a pile of toast in one go, you'll eat it. If you have to go to the bother of making it one slice at a time you'll definitely eat less.

Another absolute rule should be to keep serving-dishes away from the table. You won't have the same temptation to have further helpings. In the same way you should dispose of all leftovers as soon as possible and that includes children's leftovers. If its useable at another meal put it in a container and away in the fridge, or even better, the freezer. If it is not, throw it in the dustbin immediately.

When you have chocolate (remember, you can have ANYTHING just as long as you really want it) have 'a' chocolate. Take one or two out of the box then put the box away out of sight. Nibble the chocolate, savour it and concentrate upon it. If you leave an open box in front of you it's amazing how fast it disappears without you even being aware. MINDLESS CALORIES.

Watch other people eat

Some people eat very quickly. They don't stop between mouthfuls, they chew only a short time. They start the next course as soon as the previous one is finished. They eat everything on their plate indiscriminately.

Others eat slowly. They put their knife and fork down between mouthfuls. They chew thoroughly. They cut up their food into small pieces and, as a result, it looks substantial on their plate. They have no hesitation in stopping eating when they don't feel hungry. They will leave food on their plates. They realise that if they don't 'waste it – they will only waist it'.

Eat just a little bit less

If we can register one fact throughout the Uni-Vite programme, it is that maintaining an attractive figure and a healthy body is the result of making several small changes. By far the easiest is: 'eat just a little bit less'.

If you burn up 2,100 calories a day – (the average woman probably does) – and you eat just 5% less, that's 1/20th less of everything. You take in 105 less calories a day. You won't notice the difference that day, either in the amount of food or in your weight. Nor will you notice the difference at the end of the week. You probably won't notice much difference at the end of the month either. But over a year you could have saved 10 lb. in weight.

126

New research shows just how crucial it is for the person who has lost weight to permanently reduce her calorie intake. Professor Jequier at the University of Lausanne, for instance, has shown that the metabolic rate of people who have lost 40 lb. drops by at least 320 calories a day. On average you need to reduce your calorie daily intake by about 8 calories for every 1 lb. of weight you have lost. No wonder so many people put the weight back on. The hard truth is that you do need to cut your calorie intake *permanently* compared with your calorie (food) intake before you lost your weight.

Call a friend

If you are already on the Uni-Vite programme you already have an Advisor – the person from whom you received The Micro Diet and The Micro Meal. The purchase price includes the cost of help, support and encouragement. If you feel you need help – call a friend. Slimming can be a social activity. Which is why Uni-Vite meetings are held all over the country.

Cooking

In preparing this book we interviewed a friend who had a weight problem. She was cooking. We were discussing the idea of recording everything she ate for a day, because she claimed she really ate 'very little'. Next day she handed us the sheet. She'd quite forgotten the fact she tasted three different foods at precisely the time we were discussing the diary! If you need to taste, use a teaspoon and the smallest piece.

Preparing Food

How often have you put out 'nibbles' before a party – crisps, peanuts, dips, snacks – and found you'd eaten half a plateful just by picking at them each time you walked past? So put them away till the last minute. Equally, after the party, put leftovers away immediately.

127

Eating Out

At a party, most of us tend to be a little shy. Eating something can be a way of occupying our hands. Reduce the temptation by deliberately standing away from the snacks table. You can make every other drink a slim-line drink. You are still drinking, but not so much and no one will notice.

Boredom

Probably the slimmer's single worst enemy is boredom. You're watching TV and you pop a few peanuts in your mouth. (Ever tried eating just one?) Peanuts are 5 calories EACH! One packet of crisps is over 150 calories.

Hopefully your reaction to these rather disturbing few facts about the snack industry is glazed shock. In which case why not pour yourself a glass of 1-calorie soft drink and ponder on the error of other people's ways?

If vague visions of a sandwich or the now despised crisp packet continue to disturb your virtuous thoughts, we ask you to do the following, just once. Get up and go for a walk. Say to yourself, by all means, that you are only doing it to prove us wrong. But when you come back we guarantee you'll feel refreshed, in better spirit and you may no longer feel hungry. Remember the feeling and next time you'll go for a walk, not to humour our suggestions, but because you actually found it enjoyable.

If you binge – don't worry

Now here is a change you never expected! The fact is that we become overweight because of many months (or years) of eating too much – largely the result of some bad habits and poor food choices. You certainly didn't become fat overnight.

NOR can you put it all back overnight. The absolute fact is that it takes 3,500 calories to produce 1 lb. of fat. So if you gorge yourself on a whole Black Forest gateau you'll probably put on 1 lb. Now because carbohydrates can cause water retention it will weigh the next day or so like 3 to 4 lb., but no further dramatic increase in weight will occur once the body's carbohydrate stores have been filled.

So don't think all is lost. It's just a temporary hiccup in the long-term road to success. If you let one minor lapse put you off the guaranteed route to success you're being very short sighted. What you are now doing is laying down a set of life-time habits. One relapse will make no difference at all.

The same principle applies to eating out. If a friend has invited you out to dine and has put real effort into the meal, or you have a dinner date in a restaurant it is positively churlish to make a big production about sticking rigidly to a diet. Have something of everything but you can be sensible. You can choose the least fattening elements. You can eat small portions of the dessert. That way you emphasise to your subconscious that you are in control. You can have it if you really want it – and this time you decided you really *did* want it!

In fact, if you're using Uni-Vite 'sole source', your calorie intake is so small that you can afford a lapse and probably still be well under your daily calorie expenditure. However, as we've said, eating extra carbohydrates may cause water retention and a weight gain (or slow down in weight loss) that is out of proportion to the actual calories consumed. This is why it is really worth sticking faithfully to the exact programme.

Listening to your body

We often use this phrase. It means allowing time to let your body tell you what it wants. Now this doesn't just mean being aware when you are full!

Sometimes your body seems to cry out for particular foods. If you have a larder full of healthy foods and a fridge full of raw vegetables and fruit juices, and you still crave for a quarter pounder, you should eat it! No type of food is forbidden in the Uni-Vite Programme. There is a

129

sound practical reason. Let's suppose you really fancy a big helping of that trifle in the fridge. Your sensible self says – 'Are you mad? There must be 700 calories in that trifle!' But the craving persists. 'You'd be far better off with a nice raw carrot and a celery snack,' says your rational self. But the urge for trifle persists. So you try to silence it by eating a banana. But the craving is still there!

Well, you've guessed. In the end you have the trifle. So now you've had the raw vegetable and the banana and the trifle! You might as well have had a small piece of the trifle at the beginning! Denying yourself is only continuing with old style dieting mentality – and that's failed millions of times.

So is nothing forbidden? Not even the 'naughty food' – chocolates for example? No, chocolates if you really want them are OK. The reason is that if something is forbidden, that's half its attraction! When you can have it, it loses some of its glamour. And it loses some of its glamour when we know why it is such a poor food choice.

When you know the full effect some foods have on you – high-sugar foods for example – you can never really feel the same about them. You truly can lose your taste for foods on which you previously binged.

Make a start – forget the old style diet mentality

The reason diets fail is that they ask you to make too many changes too fast. The 'all or nothing' approach nearly always ends up as 'nothing'. The whole theme of the Uni-Vite Programme of Keeping Slim is that it is a series of individually minor changes that add up to success. None of the individual changes involves much effort, but together they accumulate to a major and decisive change.

The first thing that's wrong with old style diets is that they emphasise 'Don't!' If you are told not to do something – what is the very thing that you start thinking about?

A friend of ours gave up smoking in ONE day. When

we asked him whether he had stopped smoking he very revealingly answered: 'No. I can have a cigarette anytime I want – but I don't really want one just at the moment.' He wasn't denying himself, he wasn't exercising 'will power', which involves concentrating on the very thing he wanted to forget. He was simply making the key statement: 'I can have it if I want it – but I don't really want it.'

There is an absolutely crucial difference in attitude here. The typical old style dieter will deny himself. Do without breakfast and skip lunch. So far he feels virtuous. But then, once home, he is feeling desperately hungry. So food begins to loom large in his mind. In an entirely mistaken impression that he is exercising will power, he tries to resist eating. So by the time he does start to eat, you can bet he'll eat the wrong foods, and too fast. In the end he'll eat far more than he ever would have done with a more relaxed approach. The likely result is that he'll then feel overfed, guilty and quite possibly abandon the whole thing as not worthwhile. That vicious circle all started because he started with the old style diet mentality – concentrating on what NOT to do. Using misguided will power instead of common sense.

In contrast, we believe the ONLY way to succeed is to acknowledge that food is there to be enjoyed and 'you can have it if you really want it'. But there is the rub! Do you *really* want it? Now clearly you must be willing to answer the question realistically. If you ask the question while you're holding a second helping of chocolate cake in your hand the answer is rather likely to be 'yes'! You need to be able to answer the question under more objective circum-stances. For example:

1. **You are at the table**. Do you really want an extra helping? Wait five minutes. Be aware of how your body feels. Then answer. If you still want more, go ahead and enjoy it. You decided consciously to eat it rather than automatically starting on the second helping – and you should relish it.

2. **You walk into the kitchen and see some leftover cake**. Don't just grab it. You can have it if you really want it but

do you really want it? Walk out again and do something for the next ten minutes. Now decide.

3. **You are at a restaurant**. The waiter asks if you want dessert. Remember you can have it if you really want it. Say you'll let him know in a minute or two. Get up from the table and go to the cloakroom.

Now you are removed from the environment when the automatic unthinking reaction is to continue with a sweet. Given the short break you will now probably become aware that you actually feel pretty full. There is a good chance when you return to the table you can genuinely say, 'No, on reflection I really don't want a dessert.'

4. **You are relaxing in the evening and you fancy some chocolate**. A few squares is hardly a disaster, so you can have it if you really want it. Now if you've been taking note of the advice in this book, there will be none in the house. (Because if it isn't immediately available you can't immediately eat it.) So now the question is, 'Do I really want it – and do I want it enough to walk down to the shop or off-licence for it?' That's an instructive question!

5. **You are at home at the weekend and you fancy a snack of hamburgers and chips**. Fair enough. You know enough to grill the quarter pounder rather than fry it – and to use the large chips because they absorb less fat. Do you really want it? You busy yourself and wait five minutes. The answer is 'yes'.

Now's the time to learn to be a 'calorie trader'. A calorie trader is someone who is quite happy to trade a little exercise for some favourite food. So you decide that the favourite treat is around 600 calories (endlessly calculating the last few calories is pointless and boring). Walking briskly burns up about five calories a minute. So the question is – do you want the high tea enough to trade it for a 120-minute walk?

Now this question not only helps highlight the point of whether you really want the meal – it is an excellent way of making calories a meaningful measurement. It's quite fun, and definitely educational, to express food not only in calories but in 'exercise equivalents'. Why not play the game yourself, converting your favourite foods into minutes of walking. (1 minute walking = 5 calories burnt.) Here are a few examples.

	CALORIES involved	Minutes of walking to burn up calories
2 slices toast with butter and marmalade	365	91 minutes
1 corned beef sandwich	370	93 minutes
1 piece chocolate cake	232	58 minutes
1 pkt. peanuts (2 oz.)	325	81 minutes
1 pkt. crisps (2 oz.)	305	76 minutes
1 sausage roll (2½ oz.)	325	81 minutes
1 medium mince pie (2 oz.)	260	65 minutes
2 pancakes	275	69 minutes
1 chocolate bar 'Yorkie' (2.2 oz.)	330	83 minutes
Ice cream (3 oz.)	140	35 minutes
1 cup cocoa	240	60 minutes
1 pint beer	190	48 minutes
1½ oz. cream cheese and 2 cream crackers	272	68 minutes

Let us make a suggestion. Next time you do decide 'I really do want that extra', go ahead – but first walk it off. We promise you, you'll enjoy the walk, you'll feel a lot more relaxed, and you'll enjoy that 'extra' all the more.

A recap

Let's take a break and review what we have learnt.
1.   Many overweight people really do put on weight easily. They eat more than their body can currently metabolise – but they don't necessarily overeat compared with other people.
2.   Most people eat for psychological reasons as well as to satisfy their physical needs. Unfortunately, the person who puts on weight easily finds that their body just can't cope with those extra calories so they can't afford to feed their mind as well as their body.

3.   Calories certainly count. It's wise to know the foods that have a well above average fattening effect. That knowledge will genuinely influence our attitude towards them. We can cook and eat to de-emphasise them.

4.   Old style dieting and denial is counter productive. You know and we know that it is not that simple. What's needed is a positive programme that's realistic, enjoyable and which works.

The Uni-Vite 'Stay Slim' programme works. It partly involves pure common sense and partly involves putting into practice a number of minor changes. None of them is individually difficult – but they can add up to a dramatic effect on your life.

Case history

Name: Sandie Hawkins
Home town: Gloucester
Weight loss: 5 st.

Sandie Hawkins's shapely size 8 figure soared to a frumpy 16 and 14 st. in weight, when a spinal injury left her completely bedridden.

Doctors warned she might never sit up again but assured her the weight would come down when she was taken off medication. Sandie was mortified when they were proved wrong and the flab stayed put.

All attempts at dieting were a failure until Sandie (38) tried the 330-calorie a day programme. Not only did she shed those four surplus stone in just four months, she defied doctors, fighting her way out of bed and back onto her feet.

'Before my back operation I had always been slim,' confessed Sandie of Robinswood Country Park, Gloucestershire. 'To suddenly be so fat was unbearable. My clothes didn't fit, my husband wouldn't come near me and I couldn't look at myself in the mirror.

134

'When my doctors put me on a calorie controlled diet and I didn't shed an ounce in three months, they accused me of cheating. I was furious because I knew I hadn't.'

Now a trim 9 stone, the plucky mother of four enthuses, 'I feel fantastic! In fact since I started The Micro Diet I've never felt better. I've got bags of energy and I no longer suffer from bad headaches or crippling period pains. I'll never stop taking Uni-Vite. It has completely changed my eating habits – i.e. I can't face chips or fried foods. I shall always take Uni-Vite for nutrition. In fact my doctor insists on it!

11

THE UNI-VITE MENU PLAN

It is extremely difficult to devise a 1,000-calorie a day diet containing as much nutrition as the 330-calorie a day of Uni-Vite – The Micro Diet.

Over the course of a week, however, the following unique menu plan devised by Uni-Vite's staff dietitians, is calculated to provide the required amounts of vital nutrients as recommended by health authorities. The menu plan is devised to provide not only the necessary protein and fibre but every *single* vitamin, mineral and trace element you need over the course of a week. The same 50 plus vital nutrients are miniaturised into The Micro Diet formula providing all the recommended amounts on a daily basis – a task virtually impossible with low-calorie meals of conventional food.

Total days can obviously be inter-changed but try to consume the whole of the menu plan during the course of a week as this has been carefully balanced to give you maximum nutritional value in controlled calorie levels. Each day is 1,000 calories or less. The main meal of the day can also be effectively used during the 'Add-a-Meal' week of the 'sole source' plan. For weight maintenance purposes, 1,000 calories a day may be too low for many people. Therefore complex carbohydrate should be added in the form of wholemeal bread, potatoes and whole grain cereals.

Sunday

Today's calorie count 912 calories per person.

Breakfast   1 glass Uni-Vite 330

Lunch   60 g/2–3 oz. roast beef
               60 g/2–3 oz. boiled carrots
               60 g/2–3 oz. boiled spinach
               100 g/4 oz. creamed potato

Sweet   *Caribbean Banana* (serves 4)
               4 medium sized bananas
               75 ml/6 tbs. unsweetened orange juice
               50 g/2 oz. sultanas
               20 ml/4 tsp. rum

               1. Peel and slice bananas and place in
                  ovenproof dish.
               2. Add remaining ingredients to dish and toss
                  together gently so pieces are covered in
                  juice.
               3. Cover with lid or foil.
               4. Bake at 180°C/350°F/Gas Mark 4 for 15–20
                  mins.
                  Serve immediately.

Tea   *Cheese and Tomato Sandwich*
               2 slices wholemeal bread
               Low-fat spread
               50 g/2 oz. Edam cheese
               50 g/2 oz. tomato

For Tea and Coffee 150 ml/¼ pt. skimmed milk.

Monday

Today's calorie count 819 calories per person.

Breakfast 1 glass Uni-Vite 330

Lunch   60 g/2–3 oz. cold roast beef
Bean Salad (serves 4)
1 medium onion – peeled and chopped
2 ripe tomatoes
450 g/15 oz. can red kidney beans – drained
1 stick celery – chopped
1 tbs. parsley – chopped
Salt and pepper
French dressing (2 × 15 ml/2 tbs. oil, 4 × 15 ml/4 tbs. vinegar, seasoning)

1. Simmer onions until just tender in salted water.
2. Scald tomatoes and remove peel. Remove seeds and core. Cut flesh into slices.
3. Make up french dressing.
4. Put beans, onion, tomatoes, parsley and seasoning in bowl and pour over dressing. Mix well.

Evening meal *Cod with Piquant Sauce* (serves 4)
4 × 175 g/6 oz. cod steaks
284 g/2 cartons natural yoghurt
4 × 5 ml/4 tsp. cornflour
4 × 15 ml/4 tsp. lemon juice
Salt and pepper
1 × 5 ml/1 tsp. curry powder
1 × 5 ml/1 tsp. prepared mustard

1. Wrap fish in foil and bake at 160°C/325°F/Gas Mark 3 for 20 minutes.
2. Mix cornflour with 1 × 15 ml/1 tbs. yoghurt.
3. Warm remaining ingredients gently and bring to the boil.
4. Add the cornflour mixture and stir constantly and cook for a further minute.
5. Serve fish with sauce poured over.

Serve with 120 g/4 oz. boiled potatoes
90 g/3 oz. boiled frozen peas
60 g/2–3 oz. boiled broccoli
60 g/2 oz. grilled tomato

For Tea and Coffee 150 ml/¼ pt. skimmed milk.

Tuesday

Today's calorie count 941 calories per person.

Breakfast *Scrambled Egg*
1 egg
7 g/¼ oz. butter
1 × 15 ml/1 tbs. skimmed milk
1 slice wholemeal toast
Low-fat spread
Small glass unsweetened orange juice

Lunch 1 glass Uni-Vite 330

Evening meal *100 g/4 oz. lamb cutlet (grilled)*
120 g/4 oz. baked potato
10 g/⅓ oz. low-fat spread
90 g/3 oz. boiled frozen peas
90 g/3 oz. boiled cauliflower

Sweet   *Chocolate Meringues* (serves 4)
               300 ml/½ pt. skimmed milk
               4 × 5 ml/4 tsp. cocoa powder
               2 whole eggs
               2 egg whites
               2 × 5 ml/2 tsp. brown sugar
               6 × 5 ml/6 tsp. caster sugar

               1. Heat milk and cocoa.
               2. Whisk whole eggs and brown sugar lightly
                  and pour onto warmed milk, whisking con-
                  stantly.
               3. Divide mixture into 4 ovenproof dishes.
               4. Bake in a roasting tin filled with enough
                  water to come halfway up the sides of the
                  dishes. Bake at 180°C/350°F/Gas Mark 4,
                  for 15–20 minutes or until set.
               5. Meanwhile whisk egg whites and caster
                  sugar until stiff.
               6. Allow custards to cool slightly before piping
                  on meringue mixture, (to cover custard
                  completely).
               7. Bake for a further 5 minutes or until
                  meringue has browned.
               8. Serve hot or cold.

For Tea and Coffee 150 ml/¼ pt. skimmed milk.

Wednesday

Today's calorie count 903 calories per person.

Breakfast 1 glass Uni-Vite 330

Lunch   *Ham Sandwich*
             2 slices wholemeal bread
             Low-fat spread
             30 g/1 oz. lean ham
             Mustard

140

Evening *Liver Provençale* (serves 4)
meal   440 g/1 lb. lambs liver
           2 small onions – chopped
           2 small red peppers – chopped
           2 cloves garlic – crushed
           440 g/15 oz. tin tomatoes
           110 g/4 oz. mushrooms – sliced
           25 g/1 oz. margarine
           Mixed herbs
           Salt and pepper

1. Thinly slice liver and cook slightly in melted fat.
2. Remove liver and place in casserole dish.
3. Fry onions, peppers, garlic and mushrooms lightly in the fat.
4. Roughly chop the tinned tomatoes and add to the onion mixture with herbs and seasoning to taste.
5. Add this mixture to the liver in the casserole.
6. Bake at 180°C/350°F/Gas Mark 4 for 1–1¼ hours.
   Serve with 120 g/4 oz. boiled potato
             60 g/2 oz. boiled cabbage.

Sweet   *Mandarin Oranges*
           120 g canned mandarin oranges.

For Tea and Coffee 150 ml/¼ pt. skimmed milk.

Thursday

Today's calorie count 958 calories per person.

Breakfast 30 g/1 oz. High Fibre Cereal
             150 ml/¼ pt. skimmed milk
             Small glass unsweetened orange juice

141

Lunch   1 glass Uni-Vite 330

Evening   *Beef Stroganoff* (serves 4)
meal   450 g/1 lb. lean rump steak
               1 medium onion – finely chopped
               25 g/1 oz. butter
               225 g/8 oz. mushrooms – sliced
               90 g/3 oz. low-fat natural yoghurt
               ½ beef stock cube
               Salt and pepper
               50 g/2 oz. tomato purée
               150 ml/¼ pt. hot water

1. Remove any fat from the beef and chop the lean into small strips.
2. Melt butter and lightly fry onion and mushrooms.
3. Add beef to pan and cook until beef changes colour on all sides.
4. Dissolve stock cube in hot water and add tomato purée and seasoning.
5. Stir stock into meat.
6. Cover pan and simmer for 25 minutes.
7. Swirl in yoghurt just before serving.

Boil 225 g/8 oz. raw brown rice to serve four as an accompaniment.

Sweet   *Fruit and Nut Yoghurt*
               150 g/6 oz. natural yoghurt
               15 g/½ oz. chopped almonds
               15 g/½ oz. raisins
               Liquid sweetener to taste

1. Combine ingredients, place in glass dish.
2. Chill before serving.

For Tea and Coffee 150 ml/¼ pt. skimmed milk.

Friday

Today's calorie count 891 calories per person.

Breakfast   1 glass Uni-Vite 330

Lunch   *Welsh Rarebit*
1 slice wholemeal toast
40 g/1½ oz. grated Edam cheese
1 × 15 ml/1 tbs. skimmed milk
Pinch dry mustard
Salt and pepper

1. Mix cheese and seasoning with milk.
2. Spread on toast and brown under grill.

1 apple

Evening   *Soused Herrings* (serves 4)
meal   4 medium sized herrings
2 small onions
2 × 5 ml/2 tsp. pickling spice
2 × 5 ml/2 tsp. sugar
2 × 5 ml/2 tsp. sweet spice
4 × 15 ml/4 tbs. water
4 × 15 ml/4 tbs. vinegar
1 × 2.5 ml/½ tsp. salt
4 bay leaves

1. Clean the fish and remove the backbone and head.
2. Roll the fish up lengthwise and place in a casserole dish.
3. Add remaining ingredients to casserole.
4. Bake at 200°C/400°F/Gas Mark 6 for approximately 45 mins or until fish is tender.
5. Serve cold with salad.

Mixed Salad (serves 4)
8 large lettuce leaves
100 g/4 oz. green pepper
60 g/2 oz. cucumber
1 large onion
4 tomatoes
French dressing 4 × 15 ml/4 tbs. oil
3 × 15 ml/3 tbs. vinegar
Dry mustard to taste
Salt and pepper

1. Slice salad vegetables as desired, and mix in a bowl.
2. Make dressing by mixing all ingredients thoroughly.
3. Pour dressing over salad just before serving.

For Tea and Coffee 150 ml/¼ pt. skimmed milk.

Saturday

Today's calorie count 808 calories per person.

Breakfast   30 g/1 oz. High Fibre Cereal
150 ml/¼ pt. skimmed milk
Small glass unsweetened orange juice

Lunch   1 glass Uni-Vite 330

Evening	*Chicken Tandoori* (serves 4)
meal	4 × 90 g/3 oz. chicken breasts (without skin)

Evening meal

Chicken Tandoori (serves 4)
4 × 90 g/3 oz. chicken breasts (without skin)
2 cartons natural yoghurt
1 × 2.5 ml/½ tsp. paprika
1 × 2.5 ml/½ tsp. ground ginger
3 × 2.5 ml/1½ tsp. curry powder
2 × 15 ml/2 tbs. lemon juice
1 × 5 ml/1 tsp. salt
1 clove garlic – crushed

1. Cut slashes in chicken pieces.
2. Combine remaining ingredients for marinade.
3. Place chicken in marinade, cover and leave for 2–12 hours.
4. Grill chicken for approximately 20 mins., using marinade for basting.
5. All marinade should be used up in cooking.
6. Serve cold.

Accompaniments for four
Green salad – 8 lettuce leaves – shredded
                    100 g/4 oz. sliced green pepper
                    60 g/2 oz. sliced cucumber
                    8 spring onions
Dressing – 4 × 5 ml/4 tbs. oil
                    3 × 15 ml/3 tbs. vinegar
                    Dry mustard to taste
                    Salt and pepper
Toss the green salad in the dressing. Boil 480 g/1 lb. brown rice and serve with chicken and salad.

For Tea and Coffee 150 ml/¼ pt. skimmed milk.

12

EXERCISE – THE DOUBLE BONUS

The inescapable energy equation is that:-

$$\text{Calories eaten} \quad Minus \quad \begin{array}{c}\text{Calories burnt}\\\text{for work or}\\\text{keeping warm}\end{array} = \text{Weight gain or loss}$$

If you eat 2,200 calories and only use 2,000 calories, you gain (store) 200 calories as fat. You certainly wouldn't notice it. If it continued each day it would be 1,400 calories extra stored as fat in the course of a week. Still not noticeable. After a month you'd have put on 1½ lb. because 3,500 excess calories = 1 lb. of body fat. Still no real apparent problem. But in the course of a year, if you didn't take action or increase the amount of exercise, you would have put on about 14 lb.

As if to add insult to injury, as people put on weight they also tend to become slower and less active, a trend that cars, lifts and all the modern labour-saving devices accentuate. What's more, the less active you are, the more tired you tend to feel and inactivity actually leads you to eat more than you would with a more active lifestyle.

In many overweight people, we now know that the mechanism for controlling metabolic responses is inefficient. When we eat, oxygen from our blood is carried to our tissues and used in the process of utilising and burning up the food. For naturally slim people, who can metabolise food efficiently when they eat, additional body heat is produced and this excess heat corresponds with the excess calories that have been eaten. This process does not happen so efficiently in overweight people – so excess calories tend to lead swiftly to weight gain. People who are already prone to put on weight tend to become less active and therefore tend to eat more. It's a vicious circle. Fortunately, you can create a virtuous circle.

The kind of exercise we recommend should not just burn off calories directly, but require a larger intake of oxygen for a sustained period of about 15 minutes. Such activity – which includes simple brisk walking – is called aerobic. It's not designed to build strength, and it isn't necessary to be strenuous, but it is designed to improve your condition. You will not find it tiring – indeed it will leave most people feeling more energetic.

The exercise has a multiplier effect. The simple and direct effect is to burn calories. As with the whole Uni-Vite programme it's the small changes which have such a dramatic accumulative effect. The following table shows the direct effect of exercise. The figures, obviously, are only average and cannot take account of individual variations in body size and metabolism or pace.

YOUR EXERCISE ACTIVITY	The number of calories you burn per minute	Suggested number of mins. per week	Extra calories burned per week	Number of pounds you could keep off each year
WALKING BRISKLY	3	100	300	5 lb.
WALKING UPSTAIRS	10	—	—	—
JOGGING	10	100	1000	15
CYCLING	7	120	840	12
TENNIS	7	40	280	4
RUNNING	12	60	720	11
SITTING	1	—	—	—

We have only shown the effect of walking briskly for just 20 minutes a day, five days a week. This is because it's an aerobic exercise anyone can do. We believe strongly that it's only realistic to expect people to exercise in a way that's comfortable, easy and above all that is enjoyable.

Moderate exercise also increases your adrenalin flow and cuts your appetite. But even that's just the start. Exercise will improve the way you breathe. An out-of-condition sedentary worker breathes shallowly. In condition, through simple exercise, your breathing gets deeper with more oxygen reaching the brain. You're more alert and creative. (The Greeks recognised this and their senators used to debate issues whilst walking in their Forum.)

Exercise will also reduce the number of heart beats per minute at rest. This eases the heart's job. Your circulation will improve and often blood pressure is lowered. You can be certain that triglyceride fat levels and, in some cases, cholesterol levels will be lowered.

We called exercise the 'double bonus' because there is a further benefit of exercise – of great importance to slimmers.

Under every curve of your body there are a series of muscles. How well toned those muscles are, determines how nice those curves look! Exercising can, and does, sculpt the body towards the shape you want. In fairness, this type of exercise needs to be done with simple weights rather than through walking – but if you want curves that are sleek, it's the way to achieve them.

We have emphasised brisk walking because it's something everyone can do – for free. Of course, with all exercise you need to start slowly and do a little more each day. Vigorous exercise when you have been totally unused to it is potentially dangerous. So check with your doctor first. Above all enjoy the exercise, and make it fun. We sometimes see joggers out in our neighbourhood, their faces set in grim determination – as if they were saying to their bodies 'take that'. That's not the exercise we recommend. You don't slim by being grim! Exercise is literally Life: your body tissues will deteriorate if you don't work at them. It's as important as washing your face or combing your hair – it just requires a little more effort.

Your main reason for considering exercise may be a cosmetic one, but the benefits extend much further. Your psychological state gets a real boost. You'll be proud of yourself when you finish your walk or exercise routine, and the hormones released by exercise actually make you feel happier. Exercise is also great for circulation. It keeps the blood flowing through the body. Motion helps pump the blood. Your skin will have an athlete's glow.

You don't have to force yourself through a rigorous, exhausting routine. You don't have to torture yourself for maximum benefit. Waking up those sleeping muscles doesn't have to be a painful experience. You can do it step-by-step. Never lose an opportunity to exercise. Park at the far side of a car park. Walk up stairs instead of taking the lift. Bend over to put on your shoes without sitting down. Wear comfortable shoes in your spare time – you'll find you walk more. An exercise programme works for you as long as you work at it. You will be amazed to see how quickly you can fall out of shape! The Micro Diet gives you the foundation for a great body by helping you remove the fat – it's up to you to keep those muscles firm and shapely.

The case to take some form of exercise that involves increased oxygen use is overwhelming. As with the whole of this book, please don't just read it. Act on it. Any exercise that increases your heart rate and intake of oxygen, and is continued for a period of 15 minutes or so, is aerobic and will help to increase your overall metabolism. Three less exhausting workouts a week is far better than one totally exhausting session. Regularity is the key. The combination of diet and exercise will have the best long-term effect on your health.

THE UNI-VITE 'STAY SLIM' CHECK LIST

DID YOU . . .

* Keep a full record of what you ate (2 days only).
* Eat at least 3 moderate size meals so you didn't become overly hungry.
* Eat slowly, chew thoroughly and concentrate on the taste of the food.
* Eat only what you really wanted.
* Stop and become aware of how full you felt during the meal. Did you listen to your body?
* Stop eating when you were no longer hungry.
* Consciously leave something on your plate.
* Eat at planned meal times only and only if you were hungry.
* Eat sitting down.
* Eat in the kitchen/dining room.
* Stop and ask yourself 'I can have it if I want it but do I really want it?'
* Take The Micro Diet at least once a day. For breakfast? Before lunch? Before dinner?
* Take some conscious brisk exercise of at least 20 minutes' duration.
* React to negative feelings – e.g. boredom, tension or upset by doing something active instead of eating.
* Consciously keep leftovers and 'mindless' calories well out of sight.
* Tell a friend or Uni-Vite Advisor about your progress.
* Do some 'calorie trading' when you consciously decided you really did want an 'extra'.
* Read the 'Easy Changes' section of the book and make some of those substitutions (grill instead of frying, use low-calorie drinks, yoghurt for cream or mayonnaise, make portions a little smaller).
* Remember that a binge is only a temporary reverse in your progress so you need not worry unduly.
* Reduce or eliminate the 'mindless calories'.
* Deliberately cut down on sugar.
* Plan ahead how to deal with a future social situation.

Sun	Mon	Tues	Wed	Thur	Fri	Sat

13

WHAT YOU'VE LEARNED

The Uni-Vite Micro Diet plan will work . . . if you act on it. So have you just read the book or have you started to take action to produce success?

You can read a book on tennis, for example, but cannot learn to play until you practise – and that requires some effort. Nor can you learn to play overnight.

We are convinced that The Micro Diet programme is the most realistic slimming plan ever developed. The hard bit is easy: losing weight in the first place, and at an encouraging pace. Most dieters, on other methods, never reach their target weight. Once you've got there through The Micro Diet, you should seize the opportunity to maintain that new physique. The Micro Diet gives you the freedom to eat that you've never had before because you can use it once or twice a day, or 'sole source' for a day or two whenever necessary. If you don't regain more than a couple of pounds, you can't regain a couple of stone. Don't allow more than a few pounds to creep back on your frame without taking action.

It is vital, though to also act on the other dietary advice we have assembled for you. Follow it and you will remain a slim person forever. Here is a check list of things you need to do. Use it and tick each activity you complete each day. You may not need to do them all but you will actually see how much of the advice you are putting into practice. Please don't think 'That's a good idea' and sidle off to the pub. Do it.

Important

You will not do everything all at once. That's the mistake of old style dieting. You can safely leave the weight loss part to The Micro Diet. This check list will get you thinking slim and acting slim permanently. Tick off what you did. Then make a new check list for next week. You'll soon see the gaps and so you'll automatically focus on doing these things next week. Remember the Uni-Vite programme is all positive dos – no don'ts.

Will you succeed?

You've been interested enough to read this far. That alone gives you an excellent chance of success. You are certain to succeed in losing weight with The Micro Diet as long as you follow the directions. But keeping the weight off does definitely require some changes. These changes will be much easier because you now understand your body better and your attitudes towards eating. Clearly, the more strongly motivated you are, the higher your chances of success. You can check your probability of success by answering the following simple questionnaire. If you respond positively to just six questions you will, very probably, succeed. If you can answer 'yes' to eight or more, your chances are very high indeed.

Check how motivated you are

I now realise that being overweight is a result of me eating too much for the way my body copes with food – not necessarily because I overeat compared with other people.   Yes/No

I know that to be significantly overweight brings health problems as you grow older. I won't let that happen to me.   Yes/No

153

I am personally too overweight for my own good, and I know it is jeopardising my health and happiness.   Yes/No

I have gained weight without really realising and I want to lose it because I think I'll look younger and more attractive.   Yes/No

I am prepared to use the 'Stay Slim' Checklist for four weeks.   Yes/No

My wife/girlfriend/husband/boyfriend wants me to lose weight.   Yes/No

I really do see now that staying slim is a question of making a number of individually quite minor changes, but the accumulative effect is really worthwhile.   Yes/No

I am going to devote time to myself. I appreciate that getting and staying slim can be enjoyable and nutrition is an interesting subject.   Yes/No

I understand what's meant by 'mindless calories' and am prepared to change the habit of consuming them.   Yes/No

I would be more responsible to my family if I lost weight and improved my health.   Yes/No

I understand now that I sometimes eat, not because I'm hungry, but for all sorts of other reasons. Now I know that, I am prepared to react in a different way.   Yes/No

I am prepared to consider one regular day a week when I just take The Micro Diet as a simple way of weight control.   Yes/No

Appendix A: Information reprinted from the Uni-Vite Micro Meal label

NUTRITIONAL INFORMATION

Typical Analysis	Per serving (33g sachet)	Per day (100g)	% of Recommended Daily Allowance
PROTEIN	14g	42g	At least 100% (1)
CARBOHYDRATE	11.7g	35g	*
FAT	1.0g	3g	*

Average Energy Value			
kJ	461	1382	
kcal	110	330	

Minerals		Per day (100g)	% of Recommended Daily Allowance
	Sodium	1500 mg	At least 100% (3)
	Potassium	2010 mg	" 100% (3)
	Chloride	1800 mg	" 100% (3)
	Magnesium	350 mg	" 100% (4)
	Calcium	900 mg	" 100% (2,4)
	Phosphorus	800 mg	" 100% (4)
	Iron	20 mg	" 100% (2,3)
	Zinc	20 mg	" 100% (3,4)
	Copper	2 mg	" 100% (3,4)
	Manganese	2.9 mg	" 100% (3)
	Iodine	150 ug	" 100% (3)
	Molybdenum	160 ug	" 100% (3)
	Chromium	60 ug	" 100% (3)
	Selenium	60 ug	" 100% (3)
	Choline	450 mg	
	Inositol	120 mg	

	Per day (100g)	% of Recommended Daily Allowance
Vitamin A	1 mg	At least 100% (2,3)
Vitamin D	11 ug	" 100% (2,3)
Vitamin E	10 mg	" 100% (3)
Vitamin C	70 mg	" 100% (2,3)
Vitamin K	70 ug	" 100% (3)
Pantothenic Acid	7 mg	" 100% (3)
Thiamin (Vitamin B1)	2 mg	" 100% (2,3)
Riboflavin (Vitamin B2)	2 mg	" 100% (2,3)
Niacin	19 mg	" 100% (2,3)
Pyridoxine (Vitamin B6)	3 mg	" 100% (3,4)
Folic Acid	0.4 mg	" 100% (2,3)
Biotin	0.2 mg	" 100% (3)
Vitamin B12	5.0 ug	" 100% (3)

(1) W.H.O. Recommended Daily Allowance 37g (2) D.H.S.S. Recommended Daily Amounts 1981 (3) American Academy of Science (4) Recommendation of D.G.E. (German Nutritional Society)
* No minimum amounts established

Appendix B: An open letter to your doctor

Dear Physician,

The Uni-Vite Micro Diet is a nutritionally complete food, known as a Very Low Calorie Diet (VLCD). It is a realistic, safe and highly effective solution to the long-term problem of obesity. Although we provide a full medical fact sheet for each patient, and the contra-indications are clearly indicated below and on the product carton, the following summary will be of assistance to you in deciding whether the regime is suitable for your own patient.

The concept

Essentially, three servings of Uni-Vite Micro Diet provide the protein and *all* the vitamins, minerals and trace elements the body needs during a weight loss regime.

A woman using the Uni-Vite Micro Diet as a sole source of nutrition, will be dieting on 330 calories a day – but getting 42 g of first class protein and 100% of the recommended daily allowances of all the vitamins, minerals and trace elements, (something many of 1,000-calorie conventional food diets in practice fail to do). We recommend a man adds ½ oz. of skimmed milk powder to each Micro Diet meal – in which case he is receiving 58 g protein a day, complete nutrition, and dieting on just under 500 calories a day. This dietary balance has been shown in clinical trials to achieve a fast weight loss (20 lb. a month) whilst specifically preserving muscle and lean body mass.[1]

You can expect your patient, male or female, to lose 16–20 lb. a month. Our basic belief is that in reality patients need a satisfying rapid rate of weight loss to provide the motivation to continue to their target weight. That the concept works is proven by a recent independent survey conducted through the University of Surrey. This showed that 94% of patients using the Uni-Vite Micro

Diet thought it easier to lose weight than on any previous diet. Not only did 89% feel fit and well on the diet, but 71% noticed a *specific* improvement in their health.

The independent medical evidence

Successful clinical trials have been conducted on the Uni-Vite Micro Diet at the Universities of Surrey and Utrecht, and with members of staff at Heidelberg and Barcelona, and there is a current programme at St Mary's Hospital, London University.

Clinical trials on VLCDs generally now encompass well over 10,000 patients world wide. In 1983 the Annals of Internal Medicine, published by the American College of Physicians, surveyed the most important VLCD studies conducted over the last 10 years.[2]

Their conclusions were:

VLCDs are extremely effective

VLCD's produce short-term weight losses of 4–10 lb. in the first week and 16–22 lb. in the first 4 weeks. Over 12 weeks, weight losses *averaged* at least 44 lb. In contrast less than 10% of patients treated with conventional dietary advice ever achieve a 40 lb. weight loss.

VLCD's are safe given the physician's approval and supervision

'VLCDs of high quality protein appear to be safe when administered under careful supervision. Evidence of this safety is provided by the results of 24-hour Holter monitoring and the fact that no diet related fatalities have been reported in over 10,000 cases.'

The survey further concluded that: 'Cardiac performance is not adversely affected by VLCDs of high quality protein – in fact it may actually be improved.'

Uni-Vite's own, and other clinical trials, clearly show no side effects of any consequence, despite the low calorie level.

Blood pressure and cholesterol levels can be lowered

Patients on VLCDs are frequently seen to benefit from significant reductions in blood pressure, triglyceride levels, and serum cholesterol. Diabetic patients on oral hypoglycaemic agents may be able to reduce intake levels following weight loss.

Side effects

'Side effects are generally mild and easily managed. Postural hypertension is common but corrected by plentiful intake of water.' The incidence of side effects is less than 10%.

Conclusion

The survey concludes that: 'Large rapid weight loss and reductions in risk factors make the use of very low calorie diets attractive.'

This final conclusion is important because the report clearly differentiates modern VLCDs, like Uni-Vite's Micro Diet, from the disastrous liquid protein diets which were grossly deficient in certain key amino acids and electrolytes, and which caused so many problems in the late 1970s in the USA.

Contra-indications

Despite the very low calorie level, the provision of adequate protein and a full allowance of vitamins, minerals and electrolytes makes this a safe method of achieving weight loss for most people. It is not recommended in the presence of overt cardiovascular or cerebrovascular disease, renal or hepatic disease, hyperuricaemia, Gilbert's disease, pregnancy, overt psychosis or lithium therapy. It should be used with extreme caution in adolescent girls.

Obese insulin-dependent diabetics in hospital care may benefit from a reduction of insulin dose.

Provided that there are no contra-indications, weight loss of up to 12.5 kg (2 stone) can be achieved with the minimum of medical supervision. Patients who need to lose more than 12.5 kg may benefit from closer medical supervision with regular clinical examinations and monitoring of serum uric acid, ECG, haemoglobin and liver enzymes (alanine and aspartate transaminases).

Summary

Prior to the introduction of VLCDs formula, it was virtually impossible to devise a conventional solid food diet that gave complete nutrition in under 1,000 calories, and that became the diet 'norm'.

Now, however, The Micro Diet formula concentrates complete nutrition in as little as 330 calories a day. It permits, for the first time, fast *and* healthy weight loss. The Micro Diet has been shown to be effective and safe, not just in theory but in practice. Over 500,000 people have slimmed with it in the UK over the last two years, with no major adverse effects reported. The University of Surrey survey shows a significant majority of doctors (71%) now give suitable patients 'active encouragement' to use the Uni-Vite VLCD.

Not all patients will need to use the very lowest calorie plan, however, and alternative higher calorie plans are provided. Whatever the calorie level chosen, the completeness of nutrition will normally ensure the patient feels well and energetic while on the diet. Most do not feel hungry, which together with the satisfyingly rapid results, greatly helps compliance.

This regime is especially recommended for patients with low metabolic rates for whom traditional slimming advice demands an unrealistic reliance on self-discipline and constant, long-term restrictions.

Main References

[1] 'Anthropometric and calorimetric evidence for the protein sparing effects of a new protein supplemented low calorie preparation'. Luc F. Van Gaal, MD, Dirk Snyders, MD, Ivo H. De Leeuw, MD, Ph.D, Jozef L. Bekaert, MD, Ph.D., Department of Endocrinology, Metabolism and Nutrition, University of Antwerp.
The *American Journal of Clinical Nutrition* 41: March 1985.

[2] 'Very Low Calorie Diets: Their Efficacy, Safety and Future', Thomas A. Wadden, Ph.D, Albert J. Stunkard, MD, and Kelly D. Brownell, Ph.D., University of Pennsylvania.
Annals of Internal Medicine, (1983) 99: 675–684.
1983, American College of Physicians.

BIBLIOGRAPHY

'Very Low Calorie Diets: Their Efficacy, Safety, and Future', Thomas A. Wadden, Ph.D., Albert J. Stunkard, M.D., and Kelly D. Brownell, Ph.D., Philadelphia, Pennsylvania, *Annals of Internal Medicine* (1983) 99:675–684.

Atkinson R. L., Kaiser D. L., 'Nonphysician supervision of very-low calorie diet: results in over 200 cases', *Int. J. Obes.* (1981) 5:237–41.

Tuck M. L., Sowers, J., Dornfield K., Kledzik G., Maxwell M., 'The effect of weight reduction on blood pressure, plasma renin activity, and plasma Aldosterone levels in obese patients', *New Engl.J.Med.* (1981) 304:930–3.

Genuth S. M., Castro. J. H., Vertes V., 'Weight reduction in obesity by outpatient semistarvation', *JAMA* (1974) 230:987–91.

Vertes, V., Genuth S. M., Hazelton I. M., 'Supplement fasting as a large scale outpatient program', *JAMA* (1977) 238:2151–3.

Thomson T. J., Runcie J., Miller V., 'Treatment of obesity by total fasting for up to 249 days', *Lancet* (1966) 2:922–6.

Duncan G. G., Cristofori F. C., Yue J. E., Musthy M. S., 'The control of obesity by intermittent fasts', *Med.Clin.North Am.* (1964) 48:1359–72.

Bollinger R. E., Lukert B. D., Brown R. V., Guevara R. W., Steinberg R., 'Metabolic balance of obese subjects during fasting', *Arch.Intern.Med.* (1966) 118:3–8.

Blackburn G. L., Bistrian B. R., Flatt J. P., 'Role of protein-sparing modified fast in a comprehensive weight reducing program', in: Howard A. N., ed. *Recent Advances in Obesity Research*, London: Newman (1975) 279–81.

Genuth S., 'Supplemented fasting in the treatment of obesity and diabetes', *Am.J.Clin.Nutr.* (1979) 32:2579–86.

Appelbaum M., 'Effects of very restrictive high-protein diets with special reference to the nitrogen balance', *Int.J.Obes.* (1981) 5:209–14.

McLean Baird I., Parsons R. L., Howard A. N., 'Clinical and metabolic studies of chemically defined diets in the study of obesity', *Metabolism* (1974) 23:645–57.

Wilson J. H., Lamberts S. W., 'Nitrogen balance in obese patients receiving a very low calorie liquid formula diet', *Am.J.Clin.Nutr.* (1979) 32:1612–6.

Contaldo F., Dibiase G., Fischetti A., Mancini M., 'Evaluation of the safety of very-low-calorie diets in the treatment of severely obese patients in a metabolic ward', *Int.J.Obes.* (1981) 5:221–6.

Appelbaum M., Baigts F., Giachetti I., Serog P., 'Effects of a high protein very-low-energy diet on ambulatory subjects with special reference to nitrogen balance', *Int.J.Obes.* (1981) 5:117–30.

Yang M-U., Barbosa-Salvidar J. L., Pi-Sunyer F. X., Van Itallie T. B., 'Metabolic effects of substituting carbohydrate for protein in a low-calorie diet: a prolonged study in obese outpatients', *Int.J.Obes.* (1981) 5:231–6.

Howard A. N., 'The historical development, efficacy and safety of very-low-calorie diets', *Int.J.Obes.* (1981) 5:195–208.

Bistrian B. R., 'Clinical use of a protein-sparing modified fast', *JAMA* (1978) 240:2299–302.

Blackburn G. L., Phinney S. D., Moldawer L. I., 'Mechanisms of nitrogen sparing with severe calorie restricted diets', *Int.J.Obes.* (1981) 5:215–6.

Zollner N., Keller C., 'A 300 kcal (1.2MJ) diet using conventional food', *Int.J.Obes.* (1981) 5:217–20.

Blackburn G. L., Greenberg I., 'Multidisciplinary approach to adult obesity therapy', *Int.J.Obes.* (1978) 2:133–42.

Phinney S. D., Horton E. S., Sims E. A., Hanson J. S., Danforth E. Jr, Lagrange B. M., 'Capacity for modern exercise in obese subjects after adaption to a hypocalorie, ketogenic diet', *J.Clin.Invest.* (1980) 66:1151–61.

Bistrian B. R., Sherman M., 'Results of the treatment of obesity with a protein-sparing fast', *Int.J.Obes.* (1978) 2:143–8.

Hickey N., Daly L., Bourke G., Mulcahy R., 'Outpatient treatment of obesity with a very-low calorie formula diet', *Int.J.Obes.* (1981) 5:227–30.

Mancini M., Contaldo F., Rivellese A., Verde F., Dimarino L., 'A practical and safe programme of calorie restriction for the treatment of massive obesity', in: Howard A. N., ed. *Recent Advances in Obesity Research*, I, London: Newman, (1975) 273–6.

If you want to try a VLCD (Very Low Calorie Diet)

Naturally, now you have formed an appreciation of the Uni-Vite diet and nutrition plans, you may well wish to experience its benefits for yourself.

Contact Uni-Vite Nutrition and the company will put you in direct touch with the nearest Independent Uni-Vite Advisor.

Uni-Vite Nutrition,
Uni-Vite House,
Station Approach,
Great Missenden,
Bucks.
Tel: (02406) 6961

The team of experts who devised the Uni-Vite plan believe that anyone embarking on this or any other diet should first consult their doctor. Anyone with more than 2 stone to lose, has a medical as well as a cosmetic reason to lose weight. It is, therefore, essential for them to diet under medical supervision.

The Uni-Vite Micro Diet carton contains the following important notice:

Individuals who have conditions such as heart or cardiovascular disease, stroke, kidney disease, diabetes, gout, chronic infections or hypoglycaemia should diet only under medical supervision. Pregnant women and nursing mothers (or even women planning to start a family) should not be put on any weight loss programme without their doctor's approval. Our Advisors will be happy to work with you to achieve the results desired. Only use Uni-Vite 330 as your sole source of nutrition for up to three consecutive weeks at any one time, and only if you are dieting under your doctor's supervision.

LEARN HOW TO OVERCOME TENSION
AND STRESS IN ONLY 30 MINUTES A DAY!

The 10 day Relaxation Plan

DR ERIC TRIMMER

Stress is one of today's biggest killers. The pressures
of modern living ensure that most of us at some time
will suffer from anxiety and tension, becoming
potential victims of stress-related disease. Dr Eric
Trimmer explains how we can recognise the first
symptoms of stress in our bodies, together with the
factors which trigger them – and train ourselves to
relax, without recourse to pills or alcohol.

* This is the first book to draw together a variety of
disciplines, including yoga and autogenics, to
produce a unique plan of simple exercises.

* The exercises are clearly illustrated and arranged in
three programmes to suit all ages and levels of
fitness.

* Just select the programme which suits you best –
whether you're a housewife, pensioner or
businessman – and in 10 days learn how to overcome
tension and enjoy a healthy body and mind!

HEALTH AND FITNESS   0 7221 8605 3   £1.95

A selection of bestsellers from SPHERE

FICTION

HOOLIGANS	William Diehl	£2.75 ☐
UNTO THIS HOUR	Tom Wicker	£2.95 ☐
ORIENTAL HOTEL	Janet Tanner	£2.50 ☐
CATACLYSM	William Clark	£2.50 ☐
THE GOLDEN EXPRESS	Derek Lambert	£2.25 ☐

FILM AND TV TIE-INS

SANTA CLAUS THE NOVEL	£1.75 ☐
SANTA CLAUS STORYBOOK	£2.50 ☐
SANTA CLAUS JUMBO COLOURING BOOK	£1.25 ☐
SANTA CLAUS: THE BOY WHO DIDN'T BELIEVE IN CHRISTMAS	£1.50 ☐
SANTA CLAUS: SIMPLE PICTURES TO COLOUR	95p ☐

NON-FICTION

HORROCKS	Philip Warner	£2.95 ☐
1939 THE WORLD WE LEFT BEHIND	Robert Kee	£4.95 ☐
BUMF	Alan Coren	£1.75 ☐
I HATE SEX		£0.99 ☐
BYE BYE CRUEL WORLD	Tony Husband	£1.25 ☐

All Sphere books are available at your local bookshop or newsagent, or can be ordered direct from the publisher. Just tick the titles you want and fill in the form below.

Name _____

Address _____

_____

Write to Sphere Books, Cash Sales Department, P.O. Box 11, Falmouth, Cornwall TR10 9EN

Please enclose a cheque or postal order to the value of the cover price plus:

UK: 45p for the first book, 20p for the second book and 14p for each additional book ordered to a maximum charge of £1.63.

OVERSEAS: 75p for the first book plus 21p per copy for each additional book.

BFPO & EIRE: 45p for the first book, 20p for the second book plus 14p per copy for the next 7 books, thereafter 8p per book.

Sphere Books reserve the right to show new retail prices on covers which may differ from those previously advertised in the text or elsewhere, and to increase postal rates in accordance with the PO.